PLAB Made Easy

PLAB Made Easy

Compiled by
K Praveen Babu MBBS
Kasturba Medical College
Manipal
India

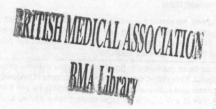

JAYPEE BROTHERS
MEDICAL PUBLISHERS (P) LTD.
New Delhi

Published by

Jitendar P. Vij
Jaypee Brothers Medical Publishers (P) Ltd
B-3 EMCA House, 23/23B Ansari Road, Daryaganj
Post Box 7193, New Delhi 110 002, India
Phones: 3272143, 3272703, 3282021   Fax: 011-3276490
E-mail: jpmedpub@del2.vsnl.net.in
Visit our web site: http://www.jpbros.20m.com

Branches

• 202 Batavia Chambers, 8 Kumara Kruppa Road, Kumara Park East

   Bangalore 560 001, Phones: 2285971, 2382956 Tele Fax: 2281761
   E-mail: jaypeebc@bgl.vsnl.net.in
• 282 IIIrd Floor, Khaleel Shirazi Estate, Fountain Plaza
   Pantheon Road, **Chennai** 600 008, Phone: 8262665 Fax: 8262331
   E-mail: jpmedpub@md3.vsnl.net.in
• 1A Indian Mirror Street, Wellington Square
   Kolkata 700 013, Phone: 2451926   Fax: 2456075
   E-mail: jpbcal@cal.vsnl.net.in
• 106 Amit Industrlal Estate, 61 Dr SS Rao Road, Near MGM Hospital,
   Parel, **Mumbai** 400 012, Phones: 4124863, 4104532   Fax: 4160828
   E-mail: jpmedpub@bom7.vsnl.net.in

PLAB Made Easy

First Edition : 2001

Publishing Director: RK Yadav

ISBN   81-7179-852-7

Typeset at   JPBMP typesetting unit
Printed at   Gopsons Papers Ltd., Noida - 201 301

I dedicate this book to my Mom, Dad and my Brother
who stood behind my dream of becoming a doctor

I would like to thank my relatives, friends and
my teachers who have enriched my life and
made me a better person

Preface

I felt completely lost in an ocean when I started my preparation for the PLAB exam when it was changed to the present Extended Matching format. But believe me, my friends, it is going to be one of the easiest exam you will ever face if you can catch the gist of the exam format and apply your concepts. The other important thing is, think only at an MBBS graduate level because the GMC expects you to think at a Senior House Officer level. The other thing which has helped me a lot is group studies and discussion and making clear cut concepts. Never waver and be sure and confident of the answer and I am sure you will come out with flying colours. I have read a lot of Extended Matching Question books, but to be frank none of them really helped me in the PLAB exam. So I compiled all the EMQ which the GMC had asked in the previous exams. These questions, are based once collection of friends as well as mine aftering appearing in the examination. In PLAB alot of repetitions of EMQ is found in the subsequent examinations. Don't spend too much time on reading big text books as PLAB is a simple exam. Believe in yourself and you are going to pass. ..Failure is not an option. ..! ! !

I wish you all the best in this world for you. ..

K.Praveen Babu

March 2001

Recommended Reading list

Oxford Handbook of Clinical Medicine
R A Hope and J M Longmore,
Oxford University Press, 1998

Oxford Handbook of Clinical Specialities
J A B Collier, J M Longmore and T J Duncan Brown
Oxford University Press, 1999

Oxford Handbook of Accident and Emergency Medicine
J P Wyatt, R N I11ingworth, M J Clancy, P Munro,
C E Robertson
Oxford University Press, 1999

Lecture Notes on General Surgery
H Ellis and R Calne
Blackwell Scientific Publications, 1998

Reference Book

Clinical Medicine
P J Kumar and M L Clark
Balliere Tindall, 1998

Contents

1. PLAB Information from GMC Booklet --------------- *1*

  i. The PLAB test Part 1 ------------------------------------ *1*

  ii. The PLAB test Part 2 ----------------------------------- 7

  iii. The First Line Investigation -------------------------- *9*

2. Extended Matching Questions ----- -------------- *12*

3. Answers -- *237*

PLAB Information from GMC Booklet

The PLAB test Part 1

The information in Annex C is valid for Part 1 examinations which take place between July 2000 and June 2001.

The PLAB test is subject to continuous evaluation and development. In consequence of this, minor changes may be made to the test as described in this annex. This annex must be understood as a general guide to the content of the test.

Introduction

Standard of the examination

1. A pass in the PLAB test will demonstrate that the successful candidate has the ability to practise safely as an SHO in a first appointment. This is the standard laid down by the GMC for granting limited registration.

Scope of the examination

2. The emphasis of the test is on clinical management and includes science as applied to clinical problems.
3. The test is confined to core knowledge, skills and attitudes relating to conditions commonly seen by SHOs, to the generic management of life-threatening situations, and to rarer, but important, problems.

Format of the examination

4. Part 1 of the test consists of an extended matching question examination. The examination paper will contain 200 questions divided into a number of themes. It will last three hours.
5. Information on how to approach the examination and some sample questions can befound on page C6.

1

Syllabus

6. Part 1 assesses the ability to apply knowledge to the care of patients.
7. The subject matter is defined in terms of the **skill** and of the **content**.

Skills

8. Four groups of skills will be tested in approximately equal proportions.

   a. **Diagnosis:** Given the important facts about a patient (such as age, sex, nature of presenting symptoms, duration of symptoms) you are asked to select the most likely diagnosis from a range of possibilities.

   b. **Investigations:** This may refer to the selection or the interpretation of diagnostic tests. Given the important facts about a patient, you will be asked to select the investigation which is most likely to provide the key to the diagnosis. Alternatively, you may be given the findings of investigations and asked to relate these to a patient's condition or to choose the most appropriate next course of action.

   c. **Management:** Given the important facts about a patient's condition, you will be asked to choose from a range of possibilities the most suitable course of treatment. In the case of medical treatments you will be asked to choose the correct drug therapy and will be expected to know about side effects.

   d. **Others:** These may include:

      i. *Explanation of disease process:* The natural history of disease will be tested with reference to basic physiology and pathology.

      ii. *Legal/ethical:* You are expected to know the major legal and ethical principles set out in the GMC publication *Duties of a Doctor.*

      iii. *Practice of evidence based medicine:* Questions on diagnosis, investigations and management may draw upon recent evidence published in peer-reviewed journals. In addition, there may be questions on the principles and practice of evidence-based medicine.

iv. *Understanding of epidemiology:* You may be tested on the principles of epidemiology, and on the prevalence of important diseases in the UK.

v. *Health promotion:* The prevention of disease through health promotion and knowledge of risk factors.

vi. *Awareness of multicultural society:* You may be tested on your appreciation of the impact on the practice of medicine of the health beliefs and cultural values of the major cultural groups represented in the UK population.

vii. *Application of scientific understanding to medicine:*

Content

9. The **content** to be tested is, for the most part, defined in terms of patient presentations. Where appropriate, the presentation may be either acute or chronic. Questions in Part 1 will begin with a title which specifies both the skill and the content, for example, *The management of varicose veins.*

10. You will be expected to know about conditions that are common or important in the United Kingdom for all of the systems outlined below. **Examples** of the cases that may be asked about are given under each heading and may appear under more than one heading.

11. *These examples are for illustration and the list is not exhaustive. Other similar conditions might appear in the examination.*

a. **Accident and Emergency medicine (to include trauma and burns)**
   Examples: Abdominal injuries, abdominal pain, back pain, bites and stings, breathlessness/wheeze, bruising and purpura, burns, chest pain, collapse, coma, convulsions, diabetes, epilepsy, eye problems, fractures, dislocations, head injury, loss of consciousness, non-accidental injury, sprains and strains, testicular pain.

b. **Blood (to include coagulation defects)**
   Examples: Anaemias, bruising and purpura.

c. **Cardiovascular system (to include heart and blood vessels and blood pressure)**
   Examples: Aortic aneurysm, chest pain, deep vein thrombosis (DVT), diagnosis and management of

hypertension, heart failure, ischaemic limbs, myocardial infarction, myocardial ischaemia, stroke, varicose veins.

d. **Dermatology, allergy, immunology and infectious diseases**
   Examples: Allergy, fever and rashes, influenza/pneumonia, meningitis, skin cancers.

e. **ENT and eyes**
   Examples: Earache, hearing problems, hoarseness, difficulty in swallowing, glaucoma, 'red eyes', sudden visual loss.

f. **Female reproductive system (to include obstetrics, gynaecology and breast)**
   Examples: Abortion/sterilisation, breast lump, contraception, infertility, menstrual disorders, menopausal symptoms, normal pregnancy, post-natal problems, pregnancy complications, vaginal disorders.

g. **Gastrointestinal tract, liver and biliary system, and nutrition**
   Examples: Abdominal pain, constipation, diarrhoea, difficulty in swallowing, digestive disorders, gastrointestinal bleeding, jaundice, rectal bleeding/pain, vomiting, weight problems.

h. **Metabolism, endocrinology and diabetes**
   Examples: Diabetes mellitus, thyroid disorders, weight problems.

i. **Nervous system (both medical and surgical)**
   Examples: Coma, convulsions, dementia, epilepsy, eye problems, headache, loss of consciousness, vertigo.

j. **Orthopaedics and rheumatology**
   Examples: Back pain, fractures, dislocations, joint pain/swelling, sprains and strains.

k. **Psychiatry (to include substance abuse)**
   Examples: Alcohol abuse, anxiety, assessing suicidal risk, dementia, depression, drug abuse, overdoses and self harm, panic attacks, post-natal problems.

l. **Renal System (to include urinary tract and genitourinary medicine)**
   Examples: Haematuria, renal and ureteric calculi, renal failure, sexual health, testicular pain, urinary infections.

m. **Respiratory system**
Examples: Asthma, breathlessness/wheeze, cough, haemoptysis, hoarseness, influenza/pneumonia.

n. **Disorders of childhood (to include non-accidental injury and child sexual abuse; foetal medicine; growth and development)**
Examples: Abdominal pain, asthma, child development, childhood illnesses, earache, epilepsy, eye problems, fever and rashes, joint pain/swelling, loss of consciousness, meningitis, non-accidental injury, testicular pain, urinary disorders.

o. **Disorders of the elderly (to include palliative care)**
Examples: Breathlessness, chest pain, constipation, dementia, depression, diabetes, diarrhoea, digestive disorders, headache, hearing problems influenza/pneumonia, jaundice, joint pain/swelling, loss of consciousness, pain relief, terminal care, trauma, urinary disorders, vaginal disorders, varicose veins, vertigo, vomiting.

p. **Peri-operative management**
Examples: Pain relief, shock, preoperative assessment, post-operative management

q. **Male reproductive system**
Examples: Scrotal swelling, testicular pain, torsion of testis.

How to approach the extended matching question examination

12. The examination paper will contain 200 questions in the extended matching format, divided into a number of themes.

13. Each theme has a heading which tells you what the questions are about, in terms both of the clinical problem area (eg *chronic joint pain)* and the skill required (eg *diagnosis).*

14. Within each theme there are several numbered items, usually between four and six. These are the questions - the problems you have to solve. There are examples below.

15. Begin by reading carefully the instruction which precedes the numbered items. The instruction is very similar throughout the paper and typically reads *'For*

each scenario below, choose the SINGLE most discriminating investigation from the above list of options. Each option may be used once, more than once or not at all.'

16. Consider each of the numbered items and decide what you think the answer is. You should then look for that answer in the list of options (each of which is identified by a letter of the alphabet). If you cannot find the answer you have thought of, you should look for the option which, in your opinion, is the best answer to the problem posed.

17. For each numbered item, you must choose ONE, and only one, of the options. You may feel that there are several possible answers to an item, but you must choose the one most likely from the option list. **If you enter more than one answer on the answer sheet you will gain no mark** for the question even though you may have given the right answer along with one or more wrong ones.

18. In each theme there are more options than items, so not all the options will be used as answers. This is why the instruction says that some options may *not be used at all.*

19. A given option may provide the answer to more than one item. For example, there might be two items which contain descriptions of patients, and the most likely diagnosis could be the same in both instances. In this case the option would be used *more than once.*

20. You will be awarded one mark for each item answered correctly. Marks are **not** deducted for incorrect answers nor for failure to answer. The total score on the paper is the number of correct answers given. You should, therefore, attempt all items.

21. Names of drugs are those contained in the British National Formulary number 37 dated March 1999.

22. Some questions relate to current best practice. They should be answered in relation to published evidence and not according to your local arrangements.

The PLAB test Part 2

Objective Structured Clinical Examination (OSCE)

Aim

1. The aim of the OSCE is to test your clinical and communication skills. It is designed so that an examiner can observe you putting these skills into practice.

Overall format

2. When you enter the examination room, you will find a series of 14 booths, known as 'stations'. Each station requires you to undertake a particular task. Some tasks will involve talking to or examining patients, some will involve demonstrating a procedure on an anatomical model.

3. You will be required to perform all tasks. You will be told the number of the station at which you should begin when you enter the examination room. Each task will last five minutes.

4. Your instructions will be posted outside the station. You should read these instructions carefully to ensure that you follow them exactly. An example might be:

   'Mr McKenzie has been referred to you in a rheumatology clinic because he has joint pains. Please take a short history to establish supportive evidence for a differential diagnosis. '

5. A bell will ring. You may then enter the station. There will be an examiner in each station. However, you will not be required to have a conversation with the examiner; you should only direct your remarks to him or her if the instructions specifically ask you to do so. You should undertake the task as instructed. A bell will ring after four minutes 30 seconds to warn you that you are nearly out of time. Another bell will ring when the five minutes are up. At this point, you must stop immediately and go and wait outside the next station. If you finish before the end, you must wait inside the station but you should not speak to the examiner or to the patient during this time.

6. You will wait outside the next station for one minute. During this time you should read the instructions for the task in this station. After one minute a bell will ring.

You should then enter the station and undertake the task as instructed.

7. You should continue in this way until you have completed all 14. You will then have finished the OSCE.

THE FIRST-LINE INVESTIGATIONS
(Results available within one hour or
have to be done on admission)

Biochemistry

U and E	(Na, K, urea, creatinine)
Glucose	
LFT	(ALT, Alk Phos, Albumin, Bilirubin)
Bone profile	(Ca⁺⁺, Alk Phos, Phosphate)
Cardiac profile	(CK, HBD - LDH 1 + 2)
Urate	
CRP	(C-reactive protein)
Blood gases	
Lumbar puncture	

Haematology

FBC	(WCC, Hb, platelets
ESR	+ simple differential)
Clotting studies	
Malaria screen	

Microbiology

MSU (Mid-stream urine)	Results available after 24 hours and only on request
Sputum	(Microscopy)
Urine stix tests	
Blood cultures and Serology	Results available after 24 hours and need second sample for stool cultures comparison

Electrocardiogram

Pulse oximetry

X-ray
Skull (SXR)
Chest (CXR)
Abdominal X-ray (AXR)
CT scan brain (as an emergency)
CT Chest (spiral CT) for pulmonary emboli on aortic dissection

PEFR (Peak expiratory flow rate)

Endoscopy
2ND LINE INVESTIGATIONS (results only available with considerable delays)

Biochemistry	Thyroid function tests, pituitary function tests (FSH, LH, prolactin, HbAIC), serum cortisone, parathormone

Blood	Differential (Blood film), bone marrow, Vit B$_{12}$, folate and ferritin
Microbiology	Serology and cultures
Cardiological	Echocardiogram, 24hr holter ECG, exercise testing, angiography, isotope studies (for cardiac perfusion and function), lung function tests
Radiology	CT and MRI scanning, ultrasound of abdomen, vessels (Doppler carotid arteries) Isotope studies: • Ventilation perfusion scanning • Bone scanning • Leucocyte scanning

N.B.

However, some investigations may be requested immediately under certain circumstances

E.g:

Echocardiogram	acutely decompensated valve disease (M Stenosis)
Angiography	acute arterial ischaemia, unstable angina in spite of maximal treatment
Blood films	acute leukaemias
The rule is:	If the investigation would change the clinical management in a relevant way, you must request it as an emergency.
And:	Always discuss matters with senior colleagues if there are any doubts.

COMMON MEDICAL DISEASE PRESENTATIONS IN BRITISH HOSPITALS

Chest Pain

(Angina pectoris, myocardial infarction, pulmonary embolism, viral pericarditis, musculoskeletal disease, hiatus hernia with reflux oesophagitis)

Dyspnoea

(Chronic obstructive airways disease, asthma, heart failure, pulmonary embolism, pneumonia, 'upper respiratory tract infection')

Sudden Neurological Deficits

(TIA, stroke, infectious polyneuritis, multiple sclerosis)

Haematemesis

(Peptic ulcer, chronic liver disease, NSAID induced erosions)

Headaches
(Subarachnoid haemorrhage, meningitis, migraine, tension headache)

Falls/Collapse
(Any acute medical illness)

Acute Confusional States
(Any acute medical illness in the elderly)

Febrile Illness
(UTI and chest infections)

LESS COMMON DISEASES BUT LIKELY TO BE EXAMINATION TOPICS

- Decompensated chronic liver disease
- Acute exacerbation of inflammatory bowel disease
- Acutely inflamed joints
- Diabetic emergencies
- Arrhythmias
- Shock
- Haemoptysis

Theme Diagnosis of Infections

Options

A. *Pseudomonas aeruginosa*
B. *Escherichia voli*
C. *Staphylococcus aureus*
D. *Proteus mirabilis*
E. *Streptococcus viridans*
F. *Chlamydia trachomatis*
G. *Chlamydia psittaci*
H. *Trichomonas vaginalis*
I. *Neisseria gonorrhoea*
J. *Neisseria meningitidis*
K. *Haemophilus influenzae*

Instructions

For each of the patients listed below, choose the most likely causative organism, from the list of options above. Each option may be used once, more than once or not at all.

1. A 20-year-old woman presents with a subacute onset of lower abdominal pain associated with frequency and dysuria.
2. A 10-year-old Nigerian boy presents with a 3 month history of a purulent eye discharge and increased lacrimation. His 16-year-old brother has a similar condition.
3. A 4-year-old boy who has just started school presents with a high fever, vomiting, headache and a stiff neck.
4. A 30-year-old man presents with a fever, dyspnoea and palpitations. On auscultation a pan-systolic murmur is heard in the tricuspid area. He was previously healthy.
5. A 24-year-old man presents with a swelling in his right axilla. Aspiration yields yellowish-green pus.

Theme Side Effects of Antiepileptic Drugs

Options

A. Carbamazepine
B. Sodium valproate

C. Phenytoin

D. Phenobarbitone

E. Benzodiazepines

F. Gabapentin

G. Vigabatrin

L. Lamotrigine

M. Ethosuximide

N. Tiagabine

O. Topiramate

P. Amitriptyline

Q. Paraldehyde

Instructions

For the patients decribed above, choose the *single* most appropriate answer from the list of options above. Each option may be used once, more than once or not at all.

6. A 45-year-old man has been on anti-epileptic drugs for 5 years. He now presents with nystagmus, unsteady movements and hyperplasia of the gums.

7. A 32-year-old man on anti-epileptic medication now presents with ankle swelling, tremor, weight gain and hair thinning.

8. A 15-year-old boy who first presented with episodes of 'absences' at school has been on anti-epileptics for 2 years. He now presents with ataxia, drowsiness, gum hypertrophy and swelling of the tongue.

9. A 15-year-old boy was treated for status epilepticus with intramuscular anti-epileptics now presents with a sterile abcess at the site of injection.

10. A 12-year-old girl diagnosed with west syndrome (Infantile spasms) has been on anti-epileptics for 3 months now presents with diplopia and nausea. She is found to have marked visual field defects.

11. A 20-year-old woman is on treatment for epilepsy. A full blood count shows the following MCV-110fl MCHC-27g/dl

12. A 34-year-old on treatment for epilepsy complains of anorexia and nausea and general fatigue. He has no body swelling. Blood investigations show Na+=124 mmol/L K+ = 4 mmol/L. Plasma osmolality is 200 mmol/kg.

13. A 34-year-old woman, with given values suggesting acute renal failure.

Theme Transmission of Disease

Options

A. Brucellosis
B. *Staphylococcus aureus*
C. *Escherichia Coli*
D. *Klebsiella pneumoniae*
E. Hepatitis C
F. *Pseudomonas aeruginosa*
G. Neisseria meningitis
H. Typhoid
I. Toxoplasmosis
J. Hepatitis A
K. Hepatitis B
L. Scabies
M. Tuberculosis

Instructions

For each of the conditions below ,choose the most likely answer from the list of options above. Each option may be used once,more than once or not atall.

14. A 45-year-old sheep farmer complains of headache, anorexia, muscle and joint pain. He has as 'undulating' fever.
15. It's a skin to skin contact disease.
16. A 32-year-old woman presents with dysuria, swinging fever and loin pain.
17. It's spread by faecal-oral route.
18. It's spread by oro-faecal route.
19. A 67-year-old man has lost 10 kg in weight, over the last 6 months. In addition he has a 5 month history of a productive cough.

Theme Immediate Investigations of the Unconscious Patient

Options

A. Arterial blood gases

B. Blood carbon monoxide

C. Blood culture

D. Blood glucose

E. Blood paracetamol level

F. Blood salicyclate

G. Chest X-ray

H. Computed tomography scan

I. Electrocardiogram (ECG)

J. Lumbar puncture

K. Serum osmolality

L. Skull X-ray

M. Temperature

Instructions

For each patient described below, choose the *single* most useful discriminating investigation from the above list of options. Each option may be used once, more than once, or not at all.

20. A 42-year-old woman is brought to the Accident and Emergency Department unconscious (GCS = 7). On initial examination her pulse rate is 80 beats/min, she is sweating and has a SaO$_2$ of 98% on air.

21. A 40-year-old woman is brought to the A and E Department unconscious (GC = 7). On examination her pulse rate is 110 beats/min, temperature normal, BM (glucose) 4.6. She was found with an empty bottle of antidepressant Dothiepin (Prothiaden).

22. A 43-year-old man is brought to the A and E Department unconscious (GCS =7). On initial examination his pulse rate is 90 beats/min, BM (glucose) 5.3, SaO$_2$ 97% on air. He smells of alcohol. There are no external signs of injury.

23. A 45-year-old woman is brought to the A and JE Department unconscious (GCS =7). On initial examination, her

pulse rate is 100 beats/min, Sa O$_2$ 100% on air, BM
(glucose) 4.3. She is accompanied by other members of
her family who also report feeling unwell.

24. A 31-year-old woman is brought to the A and E
Department unconscious (GCS = 7). On initial examination her pulse rate is 110 beats/min, SaO$_2$ 95% on air,
BM (glucose) 4.5. A purpuric rash is noted on both her
arms.

Theme Investigation of Breast Disease

Options

A. Open biopsy

B. Fine needle aspiration cytology

C. Ultrasound

D. Reassurance

E. Mammography

F. Wide excision

G. Computed tomography (CT)

H. Magnetic resonance imaging (MRI)

I. Lymphagiography

Instructions

For each of the patients described below, choose the *single*
most useful option from the list above. Each option may be
used once, more than once, or not at all.

25. A 35-year-old woman comes to the clinic for screening
of her breasts.

26. A 45-year-old woman presents with a mass in the right
upper quadrant of her right breast. A round smooth
mass is found in the axilla.

27. A 36-year-old woman comes with a hard mass in her
breast. The skin is tethered. Ultrasound and mammo-
grapy were inconclusive. The patient wants to be satis-
fied that this isn't malignant.

28. A 36-year-old woman presents with itching of her left
nipple. On examination, no ulceration is seen, but a
scaly lesion around the nipple is observed.

29. A 23-year-old woman says she feels lumps in her breasts during the time of her periods. She also feels anxious and irritable.

Theme Post-operative Complications

Options

A. Acute tubular necrosis
B. Cardiac failure
C. Chest infection
D. Deep vein thrombosis
E. Myocardial infarction
F. Pulmonary embolism
G. Pelvic abscess
H. Secondary haemorrhage
I. Septicaemia
J. Transfusion reaction
K. Urinary retention
L. Urinary tract infection
M. Wound dehiscence
N. Wound infection

Instructions

For each patient described below, choose the *single* most likely postoperative complication from the above list of options. Each option may be used once, more than once, or not at all.

30. A 50-year-old woman underwent an anterior resection for carcinoma of the rectum one week ago. She has a low grade pyrexia (37.5°C) and is complaining of pain in the left calf. She has pitting oedema of the left ankle.

31. A 24-year-old man underwent an appendicectomy six days ago for a perforated appendix. He appeared to be making good progress but has developed intermittent pyrexia (up to 39°C). On clinical examination there is no obvious cause for this pyrexia. He is tender anteriorly on rectal examination.

32. A 69-year-old man underwent an emergency repair of an abdominal aortic aneurysm. He had been severely hypotensive before and during surgery. Following surgery, his blood pressure was satisfactory, but his urinary output was only 5 ml/hr in the first two hours.

33. A 60-year-old woman has undergone left hemicolectomy for carcinoma of the colon. On the fourth postoperative day she becomes hypotensive (BP 60/40 mmHg), pulse 130 beats/min. She has a pyrexia (38.5°C) with warm hands and feet.

34. An 80-year-old woman underwent emergency laparotomy for peritonitis. On the fourth post-operative day she was noted to have a sero-sanguinous discharge from the wound.

Theme Fever and Rashes

Options

A. Erythema toxicum

B. Impetigo

C. Roseola infantum

D. Epstein-barr virus

E. Herpes simplex virus

F. Kawasaki's disease

G. Measles

H. Meningitis

 I. Psoriasis

J. Ptyriasis rosea

K. Scabies

L. Varicella

Instructions

For each of the patients described below, choose the *single* most appropriate answer from the list of options above. Each option may be used once, more than once or not at all.

35. A 16-year-old girl, with a sore throat and fever, is found to have cervical lymphadenopathy. She is given ampicillin and gets a generalized erythematous rash.

36. A young boy with fever, a headache, neck stiffness and photophobia, is found to have a generalized non blanching skin rash.
37. A 1-year-old child with oedematous lips, a red and desquamating rash of the finger tips, is found to be febrile.
38. A 15-month-old girl with a fever for 48 hours, is admitted to hospital. Her fever subsides but on discharge develops a generalised erythematous rash.

Theme Diagnosis of a Vaginal Discharge

Options

A. Bacterial vaginosis
B. Herpes simplex virus
C. Syphilis
D. Chlamydial pelvic infection
E. Gonorrhoea
F. Lymphogranuloma inguinale
G. Candidiasis
H. Trichomonas vaginalis
I. Scabies
J. Cervical erosion
K. Endometrial carcinoma
L. Cervical carcinoma

Instructions

For each of the patients described below, choose the *single* most likely diagnosis from the list of options above. Each option may be used once, more than once or not at all.

39. A 34-year-old woman presents with a malodorous discharge. A wet smear shows 'clue cells'.
40. A 28-year-old woman presents with a white curdly discharge from her vagina. Wet smear shows mycelium growth.
41. A 32-year-old woman presents with painful shallow ulcers around the vulva and an offensive white discharge.

42. A 28-year-old woman presents with lower abdominal pain an offensive discharge and deep dyspaerunia. She has no gonorrhoea.
43. A 31-year-old woman complains of a chronic non foul smelling discharge. She bleeds after sexual intercourse.

Theme Diagnosis of Head Injury

Options

A. Subarachnoid haemorrhage

B. Subdural haemorrhage

C. Fracture base of skull

D. Mild injury

E. Moderate injury

F. Cerebral haemorrhage

G. Cephalohaematoma

H. Extradural haemorrhage

I. Granulomatous meningitis

J. Fracture of involving occipital bone

Instructions

For each of the patients described below, choose the *single* most likely diagnosis from the list of options above. Each option may be used once, more than once or not at all.

44. A cyclist is involved in an accident and is brought into the Accident and Emergency Department with a GCS of 8 and no physical injuries. On examination of the ear, there is a haemotympanum.
45. An alcoholic has had recurrent falls, presents to the Accident and Emergency Department with deterioration of consciousness. On examination, the Glasgow Coma Scale is 12.
46. Following a motoring accident, a patient is brought into the Accident and Emergency with loss of consciousness. He regains consciousness and complains of headache and is found to have neck stiffnes on examination.
47. A 32-year-old man is involved in a road traffic accident. He loses consciousness and regains it later. There are no external injuries found on him.

Theme Diagnosis of Weight Loss

Options

A. Starvation
B. Malabsorption
C. Anorexia nervosa
D. Depression
E. Hyperthyroidism
F. Atrophic gastritis
G. Dementia

Instructions

For each of the patients described below choose the *single* most likely cause of weight loss. Each option may be used once, more than once or not at all.

48. A 19-year-old girl presents to her GP before she sits for her A-level weight. She also complains ot ammenorrhoea, she's feeling unwell. On general examination no significant findings are found, but she has lost 15 kg. A middle aged lady, a company executive, has had her company recently restructured. She is divorced. She now complains of weight loss, tiredness and insomnia.

49. A 45-year-old man presents to the Accident and Emergency Department a history of diarrhoea, weight loss, palpitations. On examination there were no significant findings.

50. An elderly man with liver disease associated with chronic alcoholism. On examination, he had signs of weight loss and stigmata of liver disease.

Theme Investigation of Haematuria

Options

A. Mid stream urine microscopy and culture
B. Mid stream urine microscopy for casts
C. Ultra sound of kidney, ureters and bladder
D. Isotope scanning

E. Micturating cystourethrography

F. Intravenous urography

G. Computed tomography of the abdomen

H. Ultrasound of the abdomen

I. Cystoscopy

Instructions

For each of the patients described below choose the most appropriate investigation from the list of options above. Each option may be used once, more than once or not at all.

51. A young woman complains of painful haematuria.

52. A 43-year-old man complains of severe right loin pain and haematuria.

53. A 22-year-old university student is found to have microscopic haematuria on routine investigation.

54. A 50-year-old man complains of painless haematuria.

Theme Causes of Pneumonia

Options

A. *Chlamydia psittaci*

B. *Staphylococcus areus*

C. *Streptococcus pneumoniae*

D. *Mycoplasma pneumoniae*

E. *Legionella pneumoniae*

F. *Mycoplasma tuberculosis*

G. *Haemophilus influenzae*

H. *Chlamydia trachomatis*

I. *Pneumocystis carinii*

Instructions

For each of the patients described below, choose the *single* most likely cause of pneumonia, from the list of organisms above. Each option may be used once, more than once or not at all.

55. A homeless alcoholic with a chronic cough productive cough, presents with haemoptysis. The chest X-ray shows a cavitating lesion.

56. A chronic smoker with chronic obstructive airways disease develops a fever. He reports bringing up green phlegm on coughing.
57. A 32-year-old woman who works in a pet shop complains of fever, a dry cough and increasing breathlessness.
58. A 30-year-old woman, has just returned from a holiday in Cyprus. She complains of a dry cough, fever, malaise. A chest X-ray shows patchy consolidation.
59. A young male homosexual with Kaposi's sarcoma complains of increasing breathlessness and a dry cough.

Theme Causes of Ascites

Options

A. Carcinomatosis peritonei
B. Budd chiari syndrome
C. Liver cirrhosis
D. Nephrotic syndrome
E. Primary hepatoma
F. Hepatocellular carcinoma
G. Bacterial peritonitis
H. TB peritonitis
 I. Congestive cardiac failure

Instructions

For each of the patients described below, choose the *single* most likely cause of ascites from the list of options above. Each option may be used once, more than once or not at all.

60. A 54-year-old man with metastatic liver disease develops exudative ascites.
61. A 57-year-old man has a history of recurrent ascites which is exudative in nature. On abdominal paracentensis numerous neutrophils are found in the ascitic fluid.
62. An immigrant from India has been in the UK for 10 years, but regularly goes back to her country for summer holidays. She frequently develops exudative ascites, and has lost considerable.
63. A middle aged man presents with bilateral pitting pedal oedema, ascites, a raised JVP. The ascitic fluid is found to be a transudate.

Theme Investigation of Breast Disease

Options

A. Fine needle aspiration cytology

B. Stereotype cone biopsy

C. Wide excision

D. Mammography

E. Ultrasound

F. Computed tomography (CT) scan

G. Magnetic resonance imaging (MRI)

H. Family history

I. Ductulography

Instructions

For each of the patients described below, choose the *single* most appropriate investigation from the list of options above.

64. A 28-year-old woman who presents with a mass in the upper lateral quadrant of her breast. On examination, she has a discrete 2cm mass which is mobile and non tender and doesn't involve the axilla. She has a morbid fear of needles.

65. A 24-year-old woman presents with a diffuse nodular breast swelling, which seems to increase in size during her periods. There is no axillary involvement and it disappears after her menses.

66. A 59-year-old woman has a mass in the upper lateral quadrant of her left breast. The skin is pulled in, and there is no axillary involvement.

67. A 34-year-old woman had a mammography done. It showed diffuse calcifications. She wants to know for sure that she has no malignancy.

Theme Diagnosis of Testicular Pain

Options

A. Orchitis

B. Epididymitis

C. Testicular torsion

D. Varicocoele

E. Inguinal hernia

F. Testicular tumour

Instructions

For each of the patients described below, choose the *single* most likely diagnosis from the list of options above. Each option may be used once more than once or not at all.

68. An 18-year-old boy develops sudden pain in the left testis while cycling to school.

69. A 24-year-old complains of pain in his right testis. He also reports pains on opening his mouth.

70. A 54-year-old male complains of pain in his left testis on standing for a long time.

71. A middle aged man complains of severe testicular pain. On examination it's relieved by elevation of the testis.

Theme Treatment of Depression

Options

A. Electroconvulsive therapy (ECT)

B. Flupenthixol

C. Psychodynamic psychotherapy

D. Cognitive therapy

E. Behavioural therapy

F. Marital therapy

G. Lithium

H. Imipramine

I. No action

J. Psychosurgery

K. Hypnotherapy

L. Abreaction

M. Counselling

Instructions

For each patient of the patients below choose the *single* most appropriate treatment from the above list of options. Each option may be used once, more than once or not at all.

72. A 20-year-old first time mother presents with severe weight loss, anorexia and believes that her husband is interested in killing her and their baby son and feels completely worthless.

73. A 40-year-old man has been treated for depression for 6 months. He is now beginning to lose weight and getting suicidal thoughts more frequently than before.

74. A 29-year-old woman presents with inabilty to sleep, and aggressiveness and increased libido.Her husband says prior to this, she was markedly withdrawn, and blamed herself for their daughters death due to cancer, threatening to 'join her'.

75. A 12-year-old boy refuses to go to school because of constant failure to get grade A. He is threatening to starve himself to death.

76. A 16-year-old girl with a BMI of 16 complains of 3 month history of ammenorrhoea. She is not on the pill and the pregnancy test is negative. She wants to be a model.

Theme Alcohol and Drug Abuse

Options

A. Alcohol
B. Ectasy
C. LSD
D. Amphetamines
E. Cocaine
F. Caffeine

Instructions

For each of the patients described below choose the *single* most likely cause of their symptoms from the list of options above. Each option may be used once, more than once or not at all.

77. An 18-year-old girl is found collapsed outside *Angenoir* (a local discotheque). She has a marked tachycardia and is found to have water intoxication.

78. A medical student who is about to sit for her exams is complaining of insomnia, tremor and excessive sweating.

79. A divorced middle aged woman who is a chief executive in a bank is found to have elevated liver enzymes.

Theme Treatment of Asthma in Childhood

Options

A. As required oral bronchodilator
B. Adrenaline
C. Desensitisation
D. Inhaled long acting bronchodilator
E. Inhaled sodium cromoglycate
F. Inhaled steroid
G. Intermittent inhaled bronchodilation
H. Intravenous (IV) aminophylline
I. Milk free diet
J. Oral steroids
K. Nebulised bronchodilators
L. Oral theophylline
M. Regular inhaled bronchodilation
N. Regular oral bronchodilator

Instructions

For each condition described below, choose the *single* most appropriate treatment from the above list of options. Each option may be used once, more than once, or not at all.

80. A nine-year-old boy has a mild cough and wheeze after playing football in the cold weather.

81. A six-year-old girl with asthma uses her bronchodilator twice a day to relieve her mild wheeze. Her parentsrefuse to give her any treatment containing corticosteroids

82. A nine-year-old girl with chronic asthma presents to the. A AND E department with rapidly worsening wheeze not relieved with inhaled bronchodilators. Steroids have been given orally.

83. A four-year-old boy wth eczema and recurrent wheeze whenever he gets a viral infection has now developed night cough, there as been no improvement inspite of using inhaled bronchodilator twice each night.

84. A 14-year-old boy, with well controlled asthma, using inhaled steroids and a bronchodilator comes to the A and E. Department with breathlessness and swollen lips after eating a peanut, butter-sandwich.

Theme Non-Accidental Injury

Options

A. Elderly abuse

B. Child physical abuse

C. Child sexual abuse

D. Emotional abuse

E. Henoch schonlein purpura

F. Immune thrombocytopenic purpura

G. Child neglect

H. Coeliac disease

I. Osteogenesis imperfecta

J. Osteoporosis

K. Sickle cell anaemia

L. Senile purpura

M. Precocious puberty

Instructions

For each patient described below, choose the *single* most likely diagnosis from the above list of options. Each option may be used once, more than once, or not at all.

85. A mother 16-years, brings her baby for immunisation. The nurse notices the baby has multiple bruises along both arms and legs and is crying excessively. The house officer notices multiple fractures and that the baby has blue sclerae.

86. A 70-year-old man is receiving treatment for Alzheimer's disease. He is looked after by a 23-year-old grand daughter. He has recently developed faecal incontinence. The SHO notices bruises on both wrists and back.

87. A 14-year-old girl asthmatic is brought in to the chest clinic for regular check up. The H. Officer notices 'blue' discolourations of the skin in the back and further exam

revealed more areas with similar lesions especially on the buttocks. The mother who is Afro-carribean fails to explain their occurence.

88. An anxious mother brings her 6-year-old daughter who is bleeding per vagina. 6 months prior to this presentation the girl had a confirmed streptoccocal sore-throat infection, but is otherwise normal.

89. A 12-year-old girl with a body mass index (BMI) of 16 is brought in by her auntie to hospital. The girl has been staying with her stepmother and is found to be unkempt and smelly. The auntie is worried that the girl has taken an overdose of paracetamol.

Theme Investigation of Patient with Acute Abdomen

Options

A. Angiography
B. Arterial blood gases
C. Blood glucose concentration
D. Computed tomography(CT) scan
E. Diagnostic laparoscopy
F. Erect chest X-ray
G. Full blood count
H. Gastroscopy
I. Plain radiography of the abdomen
J. Pregnancy test
K. Serum amylase activity
L. Sigmoidoscopy
M. U/S of abdomen
N. Urgent operation
O. Urine m and c
P. Water soluble contrast enema

Instructions

For each patient described below, choose the *single* investigation most likely to assist in the diagnosis from the above list of options. Each option may be used once, more than once or not at all.

90. A 71-year-old man with a previous history of pain in his calves on walking, is brought to the. A and E Department, after having collapsed in the street. He is complaining of abdominal pain radiating to his back.

91. A 22-year-old woman presents to the. A and E Department with a sudden onset of left iliac fossa pain. She is pale and has a pulse rate of 120 beats/min with a BP of 105/65 mmHg. On examination of her abdomen she is tender in her left iliac fossa.

92. A 35-year-old woman presents with a 12 hr history of severe epigastric pain associated with several episodes of vomiting. She drinks 30 units of alcohol per week. She is tender with guarding in the epigastrium. Plain radiography shows no evidence of free gas.

93. A 45-year-old man is admitted with a history of 24 hrs of colicky central abdominal pain and bile stained vomiting. His only past medical history is an appendicectomy when he was 12. On examination his abdomen is distended, but there is no tenderness. Bowel sounds are increased.

94. A fit 17-year-old man presents with a 12 hour history of central pain localising to his right iliac fossa. He is pyrexial with tenderness, guarding and rebound tenderness in the right iliac fossa.

Theme Post-operative Complications

Options

   A. Acute tubular necrosis

   B. Cardiac failure

   C. Chest infection

   D. Deep vein thrombosis (DVT)

   E. Myocardial infarction

   F. Pulmonary embolism

   G. Pelvic abscess

   H. Secondary haemorrhage

   I. Septicaemia

   J. Transfusion reaction

   K. Urinary retention

L. Urinary tract infection

M. Wound dehiscence

N. Wound infection

Instructions

For each patient described below, choose the **single** most likely post-operative complication from the above list of options. Each option may be used once, more than once, or not at all.

95. A 50-year-old woman underwent an anterior resection for carcinoma of the rectum one week ago. She has a low grade pyrexia (37.5°C) and is complaining of pain in the left calf. She has pitting oedema of the left ankle.

96. A 24-year-old man underwent an appendicectomysix days ago for a perforated appendix. He appeared to be making a good recovery but has developed intermittent pyrexia (up to 39°C). On clinical examination there is no obvious cause for this pyrexia. He is tender anteriorly on rectal examination.

97. A 69-year-old man underwent an emergency repair of an abdominal aortic aneurysm. He had been severely hypotensive before and during surgery. Following surgery, his blood pressure was satisfactory, but his urinary output was only 5ml/hr in the first two hours.

98. A 60-year-old woman has undergone left hemicolectomy for carcinoma of the colon. On the fourth post-operative day she became hypotensive (BP 60/40mmHg), pulse 130 beats/min. She has a pyrexia (38.5°C) with warm hands and feet.

99. An 80-year-old woman underwent emergency laparatomy for peritonitis. On the fourth post-operative day she was noted to have a sero-sanguinous discharge from the wound.

Theme Diagnosis of Dementia

Options

A. Alcoholic dementia

B. Alzheimer's dementia

C. Creutzfeldt-Jakob's disease

D. Head trauma
E. Human immunodeficiency virus (HIV)
F. Huntington's chorea
G. Parkinsonism
H. Pick's disease
I. Repeated trauma
J. Space occupying lesions
K. Substance induced dementia
L. Toxin induced dementia
M. Vascular dementia

Instructions

For each patient described below, choose the *single* most likely diagnosis from the above lists of options. Each option may be used once, more than once or not at all

100. A 56-year-old man with no previous history is brought to the Accident and Emergency Department by his wife who says that he has become progressively more forgetful, tends to lose his temper and is emotionally labile. There is no history of infectious diseases or trauma.

101. A 74-year-old man presents with weakness in his arm and leg (from which he recovered within a few days) and short term memory loss. He has an extensor plantar response. He had a similar episode two years ago and became unable to identify objects and to make proper judgements.

102. A 38-year-old haemophilic who received several blood transfusions a few years ago presents with irritability and increasing memory deficit. He is unable to speak properly. He is on antitubercular treament.

103. A 34-year-old woman presents with memory loss, poor concentration and inabilty to recognise household objects. On examination she has a right handed involuntary writhing movement. There is a strong family history of similar complaints.

104. A 62-year-old patient with chronic schizoprenia presents with masklike face and involuntary pill rolling movement in both hands. He complains of chronic cough and forgetfullness.

Theme Management of
Drug Overdosage and Poisoning

Options

A. Empty stomach with N-G tube

B. IV N-acetylcysteine

C. Dicobalt edetate 300mg (iv)

D. Specific antibody fragments

E. Nevaripin + lamuvidine

F. Nevaripin antidote immediately

G. Desferrioxamine + 100% oxygen

H. Charcoal haemoperfusion in ITU

I. Increase urine output by alkaline diuresis

J. ITU

K. ITU + Propanolol + muscle relaxation

L. Flumanezil

Instructions

For each patient described below, choose the *single* best management strategy from the above list of options. Each option may be used once, more than once, or not at all.

105. A mother brings her 5-year-old son who has reportedly swallowed an unknown quantity of 'white' tablets. On examination the child is breathing deeply and biochemical results show an increased anion-gap. A blood screen reveals a salicyclate level of 8.4 mmol/L and the child lapses into coma.

106. A 23-year-old girl is brought to A and E after having collapsed in a night club. She is thought to have taken Ectasy (3, 4 Methylenedioxy methamphetamine). Initial resuscitation has been done but her temperature is now 39.5°C.

107. A 43-year-old chemist is thought to have swallowed cyanide and is brought into. A and E Department confused. His pulse rate is 100 beats/min and 50ml of 50% dextrose is given intravenously.

108. A 24-year-old male homosexual patient with heart failure takes an overdose of his medication. On

questioning he says he sees yellow-green visual haloes and his pulse is irregular.

Theme Aetiological Factors in Developmental Delay and Mental Handicap

Options

A. Birth asphyxia
B. Duchenne's muscular dystrophy
C. Coeliac disease
D. Foetal alcohol syndrome
E. Familial prediposition
F. Tay-Sachs disease
G. Bacterial meningitis
H. Klinefelter's syndrome
 I. Phenylketonuria
J. Normal finding
K. Fragile x syndrome

Instructions

For each patient described below, choose the *single* most likely aetiological factor from the list above. Each option may be used once, more than once or not at all.

109. A 10-year-old boy is getting very poor grades at school and according to the headteacher 'seems to think like a 2-year-old'. The mother also says the son has a very short temper. On examination unusually large testes are found. The boy's elder brother and uncle had similar complaints.

110. A 5-year-old girl was born after a normal delivery has been developing normally. After an acute illness, a regression of milestones has been noticed.

111. A 2 year girl was born weighing 4 kg after a labour that lasted 18 hrs in a mother of 2. She is able to stand but is yet to walk.The mother says her other child had similar history.

112. A 6-year-old boy with a birth head circumference of 29 cm and short palpebral fissure is found to be

mentally retarded. The boy's mother is on Acamprosate.

113. A 25-year-old bartender gives birth to a 2.9 kg baby boy. The baby is found to have a head circumference of 32 cm. She has had her job for the last 6 years.

Theme Decision Making in Head Pathology

Options

A. Consult neurosurgeon at once

B. iv 5ml/kg of a 20% solution of mannitol

C. Emergency burr holes

D. Urgent computed tomography (CT)

E. Discharge after check skull X-ray

F. A period of observation and discharge shortly after

G. 50 ml of a 50% solution of dextrose (iv bolus)

H. Naloxone

I. Pyrimethamine + sulphadiazine

J. Lumbar puncture

Instructions

For each patient described below, choose the most appropriate action to be taken fom the hst of above options above.

114. A 40-year-old man involved in a road traffic accident is brought to A and E. On exammation Glasgow Coma Scale (GCS) of 11 is found He is found, to have a bruise on the left temporal area.

115. A 25-year-old man is brought to A and E. He smells of alcohol. Blood glucose is 5.0 mmol/L and his left pupil is dilated. GCS is 7. The nearest consultant neurogeon is 2 hrs away.

116. A 30-year-old man is brought to A and E after a drunken brawl, unconscious. After initial resuscitation the patient breathing becomes progessively deeper and then shallower and puplils constrict then later become fixed and dilated. A CT scan has been done.

117. A 17-year-old boy is brought to the. A and E Department following a road traffic accident. He has rhinnorhoea and periorbital oedema. His GCS is 5.

118. A 30-year-old IV drug user is brought to the. A and E Department with a severe headache and confusion. A CT scan shows multiple ring enhancing lesions. The pulse rate is 60 beats/min and Blood pressure is 150/100 mmHg. He is severely wasted.

Theme Diagnosis of Hearing Loss and Painful Ears

Options

A. Acute suppurative otitis media
B. Glue ear
C. Otitis externa
D. Temporal-mandibular joint disease
E. Cholesteatoma
F. Ramsay Hunt syndrome
G. Wax
H. Chronic otitis externa
I. Ear drum perforation
J. Aerotitis
K. Furunculosis
L. Otosclerosis

Instructions

For each patient described below, choose the *single* most likely diagnosis from the above list of options. Each option may be used once, more than once, or not at all.

119. A 70-year-old man being treated for cancer of the prostate presents with difficulty in hearing. Examination of his right ear reveals numerous vesicles around the ear and on the meatus.

120. A 40-year-old complains of painful ears and also reports a history of bruxism (teeth grinding) sometimes associated with headaches. His symptoms seem to be worsened by stress and anxiety.

121. A 16-year-old girl presents with hearing loss. She admits to a months history of vague right earache associated with a purulent discharge. She now reports no pain.

122. A 40-year-old obese man presents with a painful right ear. Examination reveals a swollen lesion in the external auditory meatus. The pain is so severe and is worsened by jaw movement and traction on the tragus. The man reports no other problem, but is currently on glibenclamide.

123. A 10-year-old boy diagnosed wim acute otitis media 3 weeks ago, now presents with hearing loss. There is no ear pain. On otoscopy, the eardrum is concave, lustreless and has superficial radial vessels. Air puffed through the otoscope doesn't move the ear drum (negative pneumatic otoscopy).

Theme Diagnosis of Pupil Abnormalities

Options

A. Neurosyphilis
B. Fracture base of skull
C. Homers's syndrome + rheumatoid athritis
D. Syringomyelia
E. Myasthenia gravis
F. Holmes-Adie pupil
G. Holmes-Adie syndrome
H. Carvenous sinus thrombosis
I. Sub acute combined degeneration of the cord

Instructions

For each patient described below, choose the *single* most likely diagnosis from the above list of options. Each option may be used once, more than once, or not at all.

124. Examination of a 20-year-old male patient revealed bilateral miosis and irregular pupils. There was no response to light, but good response to accomodation.

125. On examination of a 42-year-old man, his pupils were fixed, dilated. The patient presented with chemosis and grossly oedematous eyelids.

126. A 32-year-old woman presented with wasting and weakness of the hands, associated with dissociated sensory loss over the trunk and arms. The right pupil

is miotic and in addition has shows partial ptosis. Her right face is anhydrotic and knees are swollen and grossly deformed.

127. A 21-year-old woman reports a sudden onset of blurring of near vision. The pupil is slightly dilated and there is a delayed response to accommodation and especially too, when light is shone in the eye. Her knee and ankle jerks are noted to be absent.

Theme Diagnosis of Stroke/ Transient Ischaemic Attack (TIA)

Options

A. Carotid artery stenosis

B. Cerebellar haemorrhage

C. Cerebral embolus

D. Cerebral haemorrhage

E. Cerebral vasculitis

F. Migraine

G. Subarachnoid haemorrhage

H. Subdural haematoma

I. Temporal arteritis

J. Vertebro basilar TIA

Instructions

For each patient described below, choose the *single* most likely diagnosis from the above list of options. Each option may be used once, more than once, or not at all.

128. A 27-year-old woman has a long-standing history of headaches associated with nausea and vomiting. On this occasion she presents with sudden loss of vision in the right half of the visual field. By the time you see her it has improved considerably.

129. An 82-year-old woman complains of increasing weakness and muscle pain to the point where she is finding it difficult to brush her hair and get out of a chair. She now presents with sudden loss of vision in her left eye.

130. A 74-year-old woman had a fall two weeks ago. She is brought into the A and E Department with slowly increasing drowsiness. On examination you find mild hemiparesis and unequal pupils.

131. A woman previously in good health, presents with sudden onset of severe occipital headache and vomiting. Her only physical sign on examination is a stiff neck.

Theme Diagnosis of Painful Joints Children

Options

A. Transient synovitis (Irritable hip)
B. Slipped upper femoral epiphysis
C. Congenital hip dislocation
D. Juvenile rheumatoid arthritis
E. Ankylosing spondylitis
F. Perthe's disease
G. Septic arthritis

Instructions

For each patient described below, choose the **single** most likely diagniosis from the above list of options. Each option may be used once, more than once, or not at all.

132. A 5-year-old boy presents with a painful knee joint. His mother notices the boy has started to limp. On examination, all movements at the hip joint are limited. X-ray of the femoral head shows patchy density.

133. A 3-year-old girl is brought to hospital by an anxious mother, who says the child is taking too long to walk normally. On examination her perineum appears wide and the lumbar lordosis appears to be increased. She complains of occasional hip pain and is seen to have a waddling gait.

134. A 5-year-old boy presents with a painful right hip and is seen to be limping. There is no history of trauma. The SHO in charge admits the boy and 24 hr later, the boy has no complaints, and is discharged. X-ray of the right hip appears normal and no other joints are involved.

Theme Diagnosis of Sudden Visual Loss

Options

A. Acute glaucoma

B. Cataract

C. Central retinal artery occlusion

D. Cerebral embolism

E. Cerebral haemorrhage

F. Chronic (simple) glaucoma

G. Hypertensive encephalopathy

H. Polymyalgia rheumatica

I. Retinal detachment

J. Temporal arteritis

K. Uveitis

Instructions

For each patient described below, choose the *single* most likely diagnosis from the above list of options. Each option may be used once, more than once, or not at all.

135. A 78-year-old man has had a painful scalp and headache for three weeks, and is generally unwell, complains of acute onset of blindness in his right eye.

136. A 50-year-old woman complains of sudden loss of vision in one eye. She describes the incident, like a curtain comin down.

137. An 84-year-old woman notices sudden increased visual impairment. She is found to have homonymous hemianopia.

138. A 68-year-old smoker suddenly notices markedly reduced vision in one eye. He cannot read any letter on visual acuity chart but can count fingers. The fundus is pale.

139. A 30-year-old man has recurrent episodes of an acutely painful red eye with reduced vision.

Theme Investigation of Vaginal Bleeding

Options

A. Cervical inspection
B. Cervical smear
C. Endocervical swab
D. Endometrial sampling
E. Full blood count
F. Gonadotrophin levels
G. Hysteroscopy
H. Kleihauer test (foetal cells in maternal circulation)
I. Pregnancy test
J. Thyroid function tests
K. Ultrasound scan

Instructions

For each patient described below, choose the *single* most discriminating investigation from the above list of options. Each option may be used once, more than once or not at all.

140. A 52-year-old woman has had a history of offensive vaginal discharge and intermittent vaginal bleeding over the past three months. Her last cervical smear was taken four years ago.

141. A 23-year-old woman has a new sexual partner. She has been on the combined oral combined pill for the last six years. She presents with a two month history of breakthrough bleeding.

142. A 47-year-old woman who has breast cancer and is on tamoxifen has two episodes of bright red bleeding. Her last period was when she started tamoxifen two years ago.

143. A 26-year-old woman with a six week history of amennorrhoea presents to the A and E Department with vaginal bleeding. An ultrasound scan reports "an empty uterus".

144. A 49-year-old woman presents with a nine month history of prolonged, slightly irregular periods. Clinical examination shows a normal size uterus with no adnexal masses.

Theme Management of Abdominal Discomfort in Pregnancy

Options

A. Give 500 mg stat PO of Acetazolamide
B. Do emergency cardiotocography
C. Propranolol immediately
D. Induce labour and deliver immediately
E. No treatment, observation
F. Abdominal amniocentesis
G. Give diazepam rectally after a period observation
H. 4-5g IV MgSO$_4$ over 20 minutes, then 1-3g/hr + hypotensive, initially

Instructions

For each patient described below, choose the *single* most appropriate management strategy from the above list of options. Each option may be used once, more than once or not at all.

145. A 35-year-old gravida 4, para 3+1 presents at 20 weeks with a grossly distended abdomen. She is dyspnoeic and complains of general abdominal discomfort. Abdominal ultrasound shows the deepest pool of amniotic fluid to be 10 cm and a normal foetus.

146. A 23-year-old primigravida presents at 36 weeks with abdominal discomfort and on examination her abdomen is found is to be larger for dates. She is dyspnoeic and complains of indigestion and claims the abdomen has swollen to this size within a week. Ultrasound shows the foetus to be normal.

147. A 40-year-old lady 38 week pregnant, is brought to A and E fitting. Prior to this, she had complained of epigastric pain. Her blood pressure is found to be 200/110 mmHg.

Theme Management of Cystitis

Options

A. Computed tomography (CT) scan
B. Cystoscopy

C. Intravenous urogram (IVU)

D. Long term trimethoprim

E. Mid stream urine culture in three months

F. Mid stream specimen of urine for culture and trime-thoprim

G. Monthly mid stream urine culture

H. No action

I. Nuclear medicine scan

J. Potassium citrate

K. Ultrasound of kidneys and bladder

Instructions

For each patient described below, choose the *single* best first management strategy from the above list of options. Each option may be used once, more than once, or not at all.

148. An 18-year-old woman became sexually active one month ago. She has had frequency, dysuria and one episode of haematuria.

149. A three-year-old boy has a first confirmed urinary tract infection.

150. A 70-year-old man with prostatic symptoms develops dysuria and frequency. Urine testing reveals microscopic haematuria.

151. A previously uninvestigated 25-year-old woman has her third attack of frequency and dysuria. Mild stream specimen of urine grows *E.coli* on each occasion.

152. A 25-year-old man has his first proven episode of urinary tract infection. The intravenous urogram is normal.

Theme Diagnosis of Chronic Joint Pain

Options

A. Ankylosing spondylitis

B. Erythema nodosum

C. Gout

D. Haemochromatosis

E. Hyperparathyroidism

F. Joint sepsis

G. Medial cartilage tear

H. Osteoarthritis

I. Psoriatic arthropathy

J. Pyrophosphate arthropathy

K. Reactive arthritis

L. Rheumatoid arthritis

Instructions

For each patient below, choose the *single* most likely diagnosis from the above list of options. Each option may be used once, more than once, or not at all.

153. A 73 year fit farmer presents with pain on weight bearing and restricted movements of the right hip.

154. A 71-year-old woman with rheumatoid arthritis on immuno-suppressive drugs presents with systemic malaise and fever and has redness, heat and swelling of the wrist.

155. An elderly woman started frusemide two-week-ago and now presents with a red, hot, swollen metetarsal phalangeal joint.

156. A 22-year-old male soldier presents with a two week history of a swollen right knee, conjuctivitis and arthritis.

157. A 30-year-old man presents with a 10-year history of back pain, worse in the morning, and one episode of iritis.

Theme Prevention/Health Promotion of Jaundice/Hepatitis

Options

A. Cirrhosis

B. Hepatitis A

C. Hepatitis B

D. Hepatitis C

E. Hepatocellular carcinoma

F. Infectious mononucleosis

G. Leptospirosis

H. Lyme disease

I. Sclerosing cholangitis

Instructions

For each strategy for prevention below, choose the *single* most likely disease to be prevented from the above list of options. Each option may be used once, more than once or not at all.

158. Care in the preparation of shellfish.

159. Immunisation of sewage workers.

160. Immunisation of paramedics who come into contact with body fluids.

161. Counselling for intravenous (IV) drug users to use needle exchange facilities.

162. Avoidance of swimming in rivers and reservoirs.

163. Avoidance of alcohol for six months after hepatitis A.

164. Mass immunisation against Hepatitis B, other than for the prevention of hepatitis B.

Theme Causes of Pneumonia

Options

A. *Bacteroids fragilis*

B. *Coxiella burnetii*

C. *Escherichia coli* (Gram -ve)

D. *Haemophilus influenzae*

E. *Legionella pneumophila*

F. Mixed growth of organisms

G. *Mycobacterium tuberculosis*

H. *Mycoplasma pneumoniae*

I. *Pneumocytis carinii*

J. *Staphylococcus aureus*

K. *Streptococcal pneumoniae*

Instructions

For each presentation below, choose the *single* most likely causative agent from the above list of options. Each option may be used once, more than once, or not at all.

165. A 25-year-old man has a three day history of shivering, general malaise and productive cough. The X-ray shows right lower lobe consolidation.

166. A 26-year-old man presents with severe shortness of breath and dry cough which he has had for 24 hour. He is very distressed. He has been an IV drug abuser. The X-ray shows peri-hilar fine mottling.

167. A 35-year-old previously healthy man returned from holiday five days ago. He smokes 10 cigarettes a day. He presents with mild confusion, a dry cough and marked pyrexia. His chest is normal. The X-ray shows widespread upper zone shadowing.

168. A 20-year-old previously heathy woman presents with general malaise, severe cough and breathlessness which has not improved with a seven day course of amoxycillin. There is nothing significant to find on examination. The C-ray shows patchy shadowing throughout the lung fields.The blood film shows clumping of red cells with suggestion of cold agglutinins.

Theme Diagnosis of Constipation

Options

A. Carcinoma of the colon

B. Parkinsonism

C. Anorexia nervosa

D. Myxoedema

E. Bulimia

F. Diverticulosis

G. Chronic pseudoobstruction

H. Systemic sclerosis

I. Hypercalcemia

J. Diabetic neuropathy

K. Irritable bowel syndrome

L. Multiple sclerosis

Instructions

For each patient described below, choose the **single** most likely diagnosis from the above list of option. Each option may be used once, more than once, or nol at all.

169. A 42-year-old woman complains of excessive thirst, polyuria, polydipsia and constipation. She admits to losing weight. Her fasting blood glucose is 5.4 mmol/L.

170. A 23-year-old man being treated for myeloma is brought to the A and E Department, confused. This followed a hour history of severe abdominal pain, vomiting. Prior to this, the patient had complained of polyuria, polydipsia and constipation.

171. A 16-year-old frail girl coplains of constipation. Her Body Mass Index (BMI) is found to be 17. She is extremely afraid of eating and admits to sticking a finger down her throat to induce vomiting after meals. She is unusually sensitive to cold.

172. A 60-year-old man with a history of weight loss, presents with bleeding per rectum. He also reports a history of diarrhoea which seems to alternate with constipation. His haemoglobin is 10g/dl.

173. A 65-year-old woman presents with constipation, and reports difficulty in starting or stopping to walk. She has dysarthria and dribbling.

Theme Diagnosis of Stridor in Children

Options

A. Laryngotracheobronchitis

B. Foreign body

C. Laryngomalacia

D. Acute epiglottitis

E. Mediastinal tumour

F. Recurrent laryngeal nerve paralysis

G. Laryngeal stenosis

Instructions

For each patient decribed below, choose the **single** most likely diagnosis from the above list of options. Each option may be used once, more than once, or not at all.

174. A 3-year-old girl with a running nose, fever and loss of appetite, presents to hospital. This was followed by stridor and cough desribed by the mother as 'barking'.

175. A 4-year-old boy presents to the A and E Department with severe difficulty in breathing and stridor. He was febrile and had a pulse of 200 beats/min. Throat cultures done upon arrival revealed a growth of *Haemophilus influenzae type b.*

Theme Complications of Diabetes Mellitus

Options

A. Hyperglycemia

B. Hypoglycemia

C. Urinary tract infection

D. Somatic neuropathy

E. Autonomic neuropathy

F. Intermittent claudication

G. Atherosclerosis

H. Arteriosclerosis

I. Lactic acidosis

J. Ketoacidosis

K. Amyotrophy

L. Diabetic nephropathy

M. Possible infection

Instructions

For each of the patients listed below, choose the most likely complication from the list of options above. Each option may be used once, more than once, or not at all.

176. A 48-year-old female insulin dependent diabetic who has been on treatment for 20-year presents with a history of 3 episodes of severe hypoglycemia. She has not changed her insulin requirement, diet or exercise pattern.

177. A 48-year-old female insulin dependent diabetic who has been on treatment for 20-year presents with urinary frequency but no dysuria or urgency. Her blood glucose is 17.5 mmol/L.

178. A 30-year-old female insulin dependent diabetic presents with failure to pass urine.
179. A 68-year-old diabetic on treatment for the last 5-year presents with calf pain exercbated by movement.
180. A 70-year-old diabetic on treatment with metformin presents with severe epigastric pain, drowsiness and confusion.
181. A 40-year-old male insulin dependent diabetic who has been on treatment for 20-year is unable to achieve/maintain an erection.
182. A 30-year-old female insulin dependent diabetic who has been on treatment develops ulcers on the dorsum of his left foot. He is unable to feel a pin prick on the dorsum of his left foot.

Theme Human Immunodeficicncy Virus

Options

A. Prophylactic AZT

B. Needle exchange

C. Refer to social worker

D. Refer to your consultant

E. Methadone

F. Counselling

G. Condoms

H. Combination therapy

I. Pentamidine

J. Pyridoxine and sulphadiazine

K. Cotrimoxazole

Instructions

For each of the patients described choose the *single* most appropriate intervention from the list of options above. Each option may be used once, more than once or not at all.

183. A 23-year-old woman has been using heroin (iv) for 4-year. She is not willing to stop using the heroin.
184. A third-year medical student was drawing blood from a known HIV positive patient gets a needle stick injury.

185. A healthy 20-year-old pregnant woman whose partner is a haemophiliac.

186. A 28-year-old haemophiliac with a history of 20 previous blood transfusions presents with a dry cough and fever. His chest X-ray shows widespread mottling.

187. A 20-year-old sexually active woman who is going to Thailand for a holiday.

188. A known HIV positive patient presents with increasing dyspnoea. The chest X-ray looks normal.

Theme the Treatment of Menopausal Symptoms

Options

A. Clonidine

B. Combined hormone replacement therapy (HRT)

C. Hypnotic preparations

D. Mineral supplements

E. Oestrogen only HRT

F. Psychological support

G. Referral to psychiatrist

H. Regular exercise

I. Vaginal lubricant

J. Vaginal oestrogens

Instructions

For each case below, choose the *single* most appropriate treatment from the above list of options. Each option may be used once, more than once, or not at all.

189. A 59-year-old woman whose periods stopped five years ago has become increasingly depressed. She now feels life is no longer worth living and threatens suicide.

190. A 72-year-old woman has experienced frequency of micturition intermittently for the last few months. Mid-stream urine (MSU) cultures have been persistently negative. She is well otherwise, but would like her symptoms to be resolved.

191. A married 52-year-old woman who has a family history of breast cancer has been experiencing mild discomfort for a few hours following intercourse for the last month. She is worried about using hormones.

192. A 45-year-old woman who has had a total abdominal hysterctomy (TAH) and bilateral salpingo-oophorectomy (BSO) for fibroids and menorrhagia complains of hot flushes, night sweats and mood swings. She has no other medical problems.

Theme Diagnosis of Renal Disease

Options

A. Acute hypothyroidism

B. Type iv renal tubular acidosis

C. Acute adrenal insufficiency

D. Central nervous lesion with panhypopituitarism

E. Cytomegalovirus disease

F. Type I renal tubular acidosis

G. Syndrome of inappropriate ADH secretion (SIADH) with nephrotic syndrome

H. None of the answers

I. Membranous nephropathy

J. Type 2 Renal tubular acidosis

Instructions

For each patient described low, choose the **single** most appropriate diagnosis from the above list of options. Each option may be used once, more than once or not used at all.

193. A 30-year-old man with AIDS presented in shock. Serum biochemistry reveals
    Potassium 6.7 mmol/L
    Bicarbonate 20 mmol/L
    Chloride 84 mmol/L
    Creatinine 160 umol/L

194. A 41-year-old Londoner developed a temperature of 41°C, 5 weeks after cadaveric renal transplantation.
    WBC 2. $1 \times 1,000,000,000/L$
    Hb   8.8 g/dl

Creatinine 177 umol/L.

Aspartate aminotransferase (AST) 82 U/L

Alanine Aminotransferase (ALT) 132 U/L

195. A 36-year-old woman with leukemia has been treated with Amphotericin B for a fungal pneumonia. She presents with muscle weakness.

Sodium 137 mmol/L

Potassium 2.7 mmol/L

Bicarbonate 19 mmol/L

Chloride 110 mmol/L

Creatinine 84 umol/L

Urine pH 6.8 mmol/L

196. An 83-year-old woman with Small cell lung cancer presents with ankle oedema and is found to have 8 g/day, urine proteinuria.He is started on Frusemide. 10 days later his Blood Pressure is 115/75 mmHg lying and 85/65 mmHg standing. Serum Biochemistry was;

Sodium 121 mmol/L

Bicarbonate 24 mmol/L

Potassium 3.6 mmol/L

Creatinine 113 umol/L

Chloride 95 mmol/L

Urea 11.5 mmol/L

Glucose 5.7 mmol/L

Albumin 27g

Osmolality 263 mOs m/L

Urine osmolality 417 mOs m/L

197. A fit 50-year-old man is prescribed oral Acetazolamide by an Opthalmologist for suspected glaucoma. He presents with lethargy and shortness of breath on exertion.

Sodium 140 mmol/L

Potassium 3.2 mmol/L

Bicarbonate 18 mmol/L

Chloride 115 mmol/L

Urea 6.7 mmol/L

Creatinine 114 mmol/L

Theme Investigation of Confusion

Options

A. Blood cultures

B. Blood glucose

C. Chest X-ray

D. Computed tomography

E. Electrocardiogram

F. Full blood count (FBC)

G. Mid-stream specimen of urine

H. Stool culture

I. Thyroid function tests

J. Ultrasound abdomen

K. Urea and electrolytes

Instructions

For each presentation below, choose the *single* most discriminating investigation from the above list of options. Each option may be used once, more than once, or not at all.

198. An 84-year-old woman in a nursing home has been constipated for a week. Over the past few days she has become increasingly confused and incontinent.

199. A previously well 78-year-old woman has been noticed by her daughter to be increasingly slow and forgetful over several months. She has gained weight and tends to stay indoors with the heating even in warm weather.

200. A 64-year-old man has recently been started on tablets by his GP. He is brought to the Accident and Emergency Department by his wife with sudden onset of aggressive behaviour, confusion and drowsiness. Prior to starting the tablets he was losing weight and complaining of thirst.

201. A frail 85-year-old woman presents with poor mobility and recent history of falls. She has deteriorated generally over the past two weeks with fluctuating confusion. On examination she has a mild hemiparesis.

202. A 75-year-old man with known mild. Alzheimer's disease became suddenly more confused yesterday. When seen in the Accident and Emergency Department, his blood pressure was 90/60 mmHg and his pulse was 40/ min and regular.

Theme Diagnosis of Anaemia

Options

A. Anaemia of chronic of disorders
B. Aplastic anaemia
C. Autoimmune haemolytic anaemia
D. Iron deficiency
E. Pernicious anaemia
F. Red cell aplasia
G. Sickle cell disease
H. Sickle cell trait
I. Beta thalassaemia major
J. Beta thalassaemia minor

Instructions

For each patient described below, choose the *single* most likely diagnosis from the above list of options. Each option may be used once, more than once or not at all.

203. A 24-year-old woman presents with a two year history of menorrhagia and complains of lethargy.
204. A 14-year-old Jamaican boy complains of abdominal and joint pains of sudden onset. He is found to be pyrexial and has recently had a chest infection.
205. A 62-year-old woman with joint deformities and subcutaneous nodules is found to be anaemic. She is taking non-steroidal anti-inflammatory agents. Faecal occult bloods are negative.
206. A 50-year-old woman with a history of thyroid disease presents with a six month history of a sore tongue. She is found to have angular stomatitis.
207. A 32-year-old man presents with spontaneous bruising and recurrent infections with marked lethargy. There is no recent treatment history.

Theme Diagnosis of Infertility

Options

A. Polycystic ovary disease
B. Endometriosis

C. Adenomyosis

D. Chronic salpingitis

E. Diabetes mellitus

F. Hyperprolactinaemia

G. Hypopituitarism

H. Hyperthyroidism

 I. Hypothyroidism

J. Pulmonary tuberculosis

K. Possible malignancy

Instructions

For each patient described below, choose the *single* most likely diagnosis from the above list of options. Each optiomn may be used once, more than once, or not at all.

208. A 41-year-old woman complains of beeing unable to conceive for 2 years despite having regular unprotected sex. She complains of sweating all the time, frequent stools and says this explains her loss in weight in recent weeks. She denied starving herself and says she has a very good appetite. Glycosylated hacmoglobin (HbA$_1$c) = 5 %.

209. A 28-year-old woman complains of infertility for 3 years. She has a low libido, and has put on a lot of weight. Her breasts are discharging.

210. A 38-year-old complains of infertility and is otherwise healthy. She had been on haloperidol treat a schizophreniform illness she had for six years. She has a healthy 3-year-old daughter.

211. A 31-year-old woman complains of abdominal pain which seems to increase during her periods. Over the last year, she has noticed difficulty in breathing and chest pain associated with occasional haemoptysis, following her periods. Her mother is asthmatic and she has eczema. She has been unable to conceive. On examination she is found to have an enlarged and tender uterus. Her Body Mass Index (BMI) is just 20.

Theme Risk Factors for Deep Vein Thrombosis (DVT)

Options

A. Dehydration
B. Hormone replacement therapy (HRT)
C. Immobility
D. Inherited clotting abnormality
E. Malignancy
F. Multiple myeloma
G. Polycythaemia rubra vera
H. Pregnancy
I. Varicose veins

Instructions

For each patient described below who presents with a DVT, choose the **single** most likely underlying risk factors from the above lists of options. Each option may be used once, more than once or not at all.

212. A 60-year-old man presents with malaise and back pain which has been present for three months. He is found to have significant proteinuria.

213. A 30-year-old woman presents with a three month history of amenorrhoea.

214. A 60-year-old man with a plethoric appearance presents with pleuritic chest pain. He has palpable splenomegaly.

215. A 70-year-old man presents with back pain and jaundice.

216. A 25-year-old woman with a family history of deep vein thrombosis was prescribed a combined oral contraceptive pill six months ago and has not missed any tablets.

Theme Diagnosis of a Rash

Options

A. Pulmonary tuberculosis
B. Sarcoidosis

C. Reiter's syndrome

D. Urticaria

E. Lyme disease

F. Dystonia myotonica

G. Herpes simplex

H. Behcet's syndrome

I. Myaesthenia

J. Dermatomyositis

Instructions

For each of the patients with a rash described below, choose the *single* most likely diagnosis from the above list of options.

217. A 29-year-old man with known arthritis presented with a painful red eye and a brownish rash on his feet. He has recently been treated for dysentery.

218. A 30-year-old woman presented to the family GP complaining of difficulty in lifting her arms up. She also reported having difficulty getting up and down stairs. A scaly, erythematous rash was noticed on the dorsum of the hand, and knuckles. She had earlier complained dysphagia.

219. A mother brought her 10-year-old son to the GP, with a history of joint pains and recurrent oral ulcers. On examination the boy had hypopyon and mild conjuctivitis.

220. A 40-year-old sheep farmer from Kent presented to her GP complaining of muscle and joint pain with an associated chronic headache, which has been present for 3 weeks. On examination, she had an erythematous annular rash with a central clear area, on her abdomen.

221. A 30-year-old woman presented with tender, red nodules on both lower limbs and forearms. She had painful joints and was febrile. She had a month's history of a productive cough and investigations revealed raised, angiotensin converting enzyme levels.

Theme Diagnosis of Acute Vomiting in Children

Options

A. Acute appendicitis

B. Cyclical vomiting

C. Duodenal atresia

D. Gastro-oesophageal reflux

E. Gastroenteritis

F. Meconium ileus

G. Meningitis

H. Mesenteric adenitis

 I. Overfeeding

J. Pancreatitis

K. Psychogenic vomiting

L. Pyloric stenosis

M. Urinary tract infection (UTI)

N. Whooping cough

Instructions

For each child described below, choose the *single* most likely diagnosis from the above list of options. Each option may be used once, more than once, or not at all.

222. A two-day-old breast fed male infant is vomiting after each feed. Abdominal X-ray demonstrated a "double bubble."

223. A six-week-old breast fed boy has had projectile vomiting after every feed for the past two weeks. He is now lethargic, dehydrated and tachypnoeic.

224. A four-month-old baby who is thriving has persistent vomiting, which is occasionaly blood stained and is associated with crying.

225. An eight-year-old girl shows signs of moderate dehydration. She has vomited all fluids for 24 hours and the vomit is not bile stained. Her abdomen is now soft and non tender. She has had two similar episodes in the past year.

226. A 12-week-old thriving baby is vomiting after every feed. He is developmentally normal and is fed by the bottle at 260 ml/kg/day.

Theme Investigation of Polyuria and Polydipsia

Options

A. Water deprivation test

B. Oral glucose tolerance test

C. Plasma calcium and ACE levels

D. Psychological and psychiatric assesment.

E. ACTH stimulation test

F. Diuretic stimulation trial

G. Echocardiography and blood cultures

Instructions

For each patient described below, choose the most appropriate investigation from the options listed above. Each option may be used once, more than once or not at all.

227. A 30-year-old woman being treated with lithium for prophylaxis against her bipolar manic-depressive illness presents with polyuria and polydipsia. Plasma osmolality is found to be 600 mOs mol/kg and urine osmolality is 250 mOs mol/kg

228. A 40-year-old afro-caribbean male presents with a swinging fever, polydipsia, polyuria and gradual onset exertional dyspnoea. In addition she has a one month history of unproductive cough and chest X-ray reveals bilateral hilar shadowing.

Theme Association of Skin Lesions and Specific Disease

Options

A. Hyperthyroidism

B. Diabetes mellitus

C. Liver disease

D. Ceoliac disease

E. Hypogonadism

F. Borrelia burgdorferi infection

G. Carcinoma of tail of pancreas

H. Measles

I. Deep vein thrombosis

J. Psoriasis

K. Leptospirosis

L. Borrelia duttoni infection

Instructions

For each of the patients described below, choose the most **likely** association from the options given above. Each option may be used once, more than once, or not at all.

229. A fit 55-year-old gentleman, complains of recurrent episodes of 'seeing visible veins on his body', which are tender. He has started to lose weight and attributes this to his diarrhoea. The consultant dermatologist thinks he has thrombophlebitis migraine.

230. A 49-year-old woman complains of itchy blisters, which are occuring in groups on her knees and elbows. The itch is becoming unbearable and she is contemplating suicide. She responds to 180 mg of Dapsone within 48 hours of treatment.

231. A Welsh farmer with malaise and arthralgia is increasingly anxious about a skin lesion which started as a papule (Diameter approx 1 mm) which has progressed to a red ring (Diameter approx 50 mm) with central fading.

232. A 42-year-old man who reports a loss in weight, presents with a shiny erythematous lesion on her skin. It's edges appear yellowish and are beginning to ulcerate with undermining. She says it started as a pustule one month ago. (Fasting blood glucose is 5.3 mmol/L)

233. A 32-year-old woman complains of palpitations and is found to have red oedematous swellings above both lateral malleoli, which she says are beginning to affect her feet. She is found to have digital clubbing and periorbital puffiness.

Theme Differential Diagnosis of Ectopic Pregnancy

Options

A. Appendicitis

B. Bacterial vaginosis

C. Crohn's disease

D. Ectopic pregnancy

E. Endometriosis

F. Inevitable miscarriage

G. Irritable bowel syndrome (IBS)

H. Missed abortion

I. Normal pregnancy

J. Pelvic inflammatory disease

K. Renal colic

L. Septic abortion

M. Threatened miscarriage

N. Torted ovarianmass

O. Ulcerative colitis

Instructions

For each patient described below, choose the *single* most likely diagnosis from the above list of options. Each option may be used once more than once, or not at all.

234. A 21-year-old woman presents as an emergency with a four history of lower abdominal pain and bright red vaginal blood loss. She has not had a menstrual period for nine weeks and had a positive home pregnancy one week ago. On vaginal examination, the uterus is tender and bulky. The cervical os is open.

235. A 16-year-old woman presents with a sudden onset of severe right iliac fossa pain. On vaginal ultrasound examination a 6 cm diameter echogenic cystic mass is seen in the right fornix.

236. An 18-year-old student, due to take her examinations, reports that she missed her period and that a pregnancy test is negative. She has worsening abdominal pain which has been troublesome for three months. She is otherwise well.

237. A 22-year-old woman who has had two terminations of pregnancy, reports that she is pregnant again. She has noted a small amount of watery brown discharge and is tender in the right iliac fossa.

238. A 27-year-old, who conscientiously uses the oral contraceptive pill, has experienced intermittent vaginal bleeding and malodorous discharge for several weeks. When examined she has pain over the lower abdomen, worse on the left. Her temperature is 39°C and her white cell count is elevated.

Theme Diagnosis of Joint Pain

Options

A. Gout

B. Pseudogout

C. Osteoarthritis

D. Infective arthritis

E. Psoriatic arthropathy

F. Ankylosing spondylitis

G. Still's disease

H. Rheumatoid arthritis

I. Reiter's syndrome

J. Felty's syndrome

K. Osteogenesis imperfecta

Instructions

For each of the patients described below, choose the *single* most likely diagnosis from the above list of options. Each option may be used once, more than once, or not at all.

239. A 15-year-old boy complains of pain the temporal-mandibular joint for three months. On examination, the SHO in Accident and Emergency notices micrognathia, loss of neck extension and unequal lengths of the boys lower limbs. Tests for rheumatoid factor were negative.

240. A 36-year-old lady presented with swollen, tender knee joints. She says they feel stiff especially in the morning. On examination, he was found to have a

temperature of 38°C and ulcerated lower limbs with evidence of hyperpigmentation. Hb 9g/dl.

WBC, platelet counts were decreased.

Albumin 20g/L.

241. A 29-year-old homosexual male presented to the Accident and Emergency Department with a markedly swollen and tender left knee. He is says its been present for about a month but has only recently become painful. He admitted losing weight and on examination a temperature of 38°C was found. He had no other complaints apart from a 2 month history of cough which he attributed to his heavy smoking.

242. A 40-year-old obese man presented with a painful and swollen ankle. The symptoms had started gradually in the previous month. Joint fluid aspiration was done and positively birefringent crystals were found. The patient drinks alcohol but doesn't smoke.

Theme Immediate Investigations of the Unconscious Patient

Options

A. Arterial blood gases

B. Blood carbon monoxide levels

C. Blood culture

D. Blood glucose

E. Blood paracetamol level

F. Blood salicyclate

G. Chest X-ray

H. Computed tomography (CT) brain scan

 I. Electrocardiogram (ECG)

J. Lumbar puncture

K. Serum osmolality

L. Skull X-ray

M. Temperature

Instructions

For each patient described below, choose the *single* most useful discriminating investigation from the above list of options. Each option may be used once, more than once, or not at all.

243. A 43-year-old man is brought to the Accident and Emergency Department unconscious (Glasgow Coma Scale = 7). On initial examination his pulse rate is 80 beats/min, he is sweating and has a SaO_2 of 98% on air.

244. A 45-year-old woman is brought to the Accident and Emergency Department unconscious (Glasgow Coma Scale = 7). On examination her pulse rate is 110 beats/min, temperature normal, BM (glucose) 4.6. She was found with an empty bottle of antidepressant Dothiepin (Prothiaden).

245. A 43-year-old man is brought to the Accident and Emergency Department unconscious (Glasgow Coma Scale = 7). On initial examination his pulse rate is 90 beats/min, BM (glucose) 5.3, SaO_2 97% on air. He smells of alcohol. There are no external signs of injury.

246. A 44-year-old man is brought to the Accident and Emergency Department unconscious (Glasgow Coma Scale = 7). On initial examination, his pulse rate is 100 beats/min, SaO_2 100% on air, BM (glucose) 4.3. He is accompanied by other members of his family who also report feeling unwell.

247. A 41-year-old woman is brought to the Accident and Emergency Department unconscious (Glasgow Coma Scale = 7). On initial examination her pulse rate is 110 beats/min, SaO_2 95% on air, BM (glucose) 4.5. A purpuric rash is noted on both her arms.

Theme Diagnosis of a Chronic Bleeding Disorder

Options

A. Von Willebrand's disease
B. Liver disease
C. Fibrinogen deficiency
D. Factor vii deficiency
E. Factor v deficiency
F. Factor ix deficiency
G. Platelet deficiency
H. Calcium deficiency

I. Normal finding in some people

J. Phosoholipid excess

K. Increased tissue thromboplastin

Instructions

For each of the patients described below with haematological abnormalities, choose the *single* most likely diagnosis from the above list of options. Each option may be used once more than once, or not at all.

248. A 30-year-old man with a chronic bleeding disorder has had the following investigations done.

Prothrombin Time (PT) 13 seconds

Partial Thromboplastin Time with Kaolin (PTTK) 40 seconds

Thrombin Time (TT) 12 seconds

Bleeding Time (BT) prolonged

249. A 42-year-old man with a chronic bleeding disorder, has had the following investigations done.

PT   11 seconds

PTTK   47 seconds

TT   13 seconds

BT   prolonged

250. A 52-year-old man is being seen by his GP for a chronic bleeding disorder and mild pruritus.

PT   prolonged

PTTK   prolonged

TT   normal

BT   normal

Factors 2, 5 and 10 are normal

251. A 29-year-old man with chronic bleeding disorder has had these investigations and results.

PT   prolonged

PTTK   prolonged

BT   normal

TT   prolonged

Theme Natural History Cervical Cancer

Options

A. 3-6 months

B. 12 months

C. 24-36 months

D. 3-10 years

E. 20 years

F. 30 years

G. 45 years

H. 50 years

I. 55 years

J. 65 years

Instructions

For each scenario below, choose the *single* most likely time or time interval from the above list of options. Each option may be used once, more than once, or not at all.

252. The time span over which a percentage of women with cervical intraepithelial neoplasia (CIN) untreated will develop cancer.

253. The age at which the peak incidence of cervical carcinoma occurs.

254. The interval for cervical smears to be taken in a woman treated one year previously for cervical intraepithelial neoplasia (CIN 2).

255. The age at which screening stops for women with a normal smear history.

256. The timescale within which the 50% of patients with recurrent disease will present, following treatment for stage 1B cervical cancer.

Theme Management of HIV Related Conditions

Options

A. IV ganciclovir

B. Emergency oesophageal surgery

C. HAART (Highly Active Antiretroviral)

D. Adjust the treatment

E. Oral acyclovir

F. Omeprazole + Amoxycillin + Metronidazole

G. Nystatin per oral

H. Vitamin supplements

Instructions

Choose the option(s) from the given list.

257. A 25-year-old gay male presents to his GP with bruises which he says are brought on by the slightest of trauma. On examination he is found to have oral candidiasis. His WBC count is 2.9 × 1,000,000,000/L.

258. A male patient with HIV presents to the STD clinic. The following investigations are done.

Hb	8.9g/dl
WBC	1.4 × 1,000,000,000/L.
Platelets	90 × 1,000,000,000/L
Mean cell volume (MCV)	106 fl
Urea and Electrolytes	Not done
Alkaline phosphatase	98 iu/L
Alanine aminotransferase	45 iu/L

259. A 36-year-old journalist has had AIDS for 2 years. He presented with a 3 week history of dysphagia, which has failed to respond to fluconazole. He was on Zidovudine 200 mg tds and Dapsone/Pyrimethamine for *Pneumocystis carinii* pneumonia prophylaxis. Endoscopy revealed a single deep ulcer in the lower third of the oesophagus.

Theme Diagnosis of Common Genetical Disorders

Options

A. Klinefelter's syndrome
B. Patau syndrome
C. Down's syndrome
D. Turner's syndrome
E. Cri-du-chat syndrome
F. Fragile X-syndrome
G. Sickle cell disease
H. Sickle cell trait
I. Beta thalassaemia
J. Williams syndrome
K. Prader-Willi syndrome
L. Di George syndrome
M. Acute myeloid leukemia
N. Edward's syndrome

Instructions

For each patient described below choose the *single* most appropriate diagnosis from the list of options above. Each option may be used once, more than once, or not at all.

260. A 15-year-old boy has very poor grades at school despite being very attentive and hard working.His mother reckons its because he is teased at school because his breasts look like a girl's. On further examination he is found to have small firm testes.He is mildly asthmatic.

261. A 5-year-old South African boy is brought to the Accident and Emergency Department deeply jaundiced. He is found to have mildly swollen, tender feet and hands. His mucosae are pale.

262. A 6-year-old Asian boy gets regular blood transfusion for his haematological abnormality. His mucosae are pale and skull is grossly bossed. Haematological investigations were done and showed;
MCHC   25g/dl
Hb   8g/dl
MCV   74fl

263. A 10-year-old boy is brought to the Accident and Emergency Department with a swollen right arm. His temperature is 38.5°C and is unable to move his arm due to severe pain. Blood culture confirms *Salmonella typhi osteomyelitis*. This is his second presentation this month and earlier presented with an acute onset hepatoplenomegaly associated with severe pallour. The SHO does a Sodium Metabisulphite test on the patient's blood which turns out to be positive.

264. A 39-year-old male is getting progessively forgetful and is later found to have Alzheimer's disease. He has small ears and an IQ score of 67.

Theme Diagnosis of Malabsoption and Diarrhoea in Children

Options

A. Lactose intolerance

B. Chronic disease

C. Acrodermatitis enteropathica

D. Chronic Non Specific diarrhoea

E. Coeliac disease

F. Ulcerative colitis

G. *Giardia lamblia* infection

H. *Enterobius vermicularis* infection

I. *Ascaris lumbricoides*

J. Hirschsprungs's disease

K. Intussusception

L. Irritable bowel syndrome

M. Endometriosis

N. Acute on chronic appendicitis

O. Endometriosis

Instructions

For each patient described below, choose the *single* most likely diagnosis from the options listed above. Each option may be used once, more than once, or not at all.

265. A 4-year-old Irish girl looks wasted and appears short for her age. The mother reports the daughter has been vomiting on several occasions in the past, with associated diarrhoea. The SHO thinks he has an enteropathy and on serology IgA gliadin and Endomysial antibodies are found.

266. A mother brings her 5-year-old son who has been passing bloody stool associated with severe abdominal pain. On examination he is found to have mildly swollen tender wrists and red nodular tender lesions were found on his forearms.

267. An 8-year-old girl has got repeated episodes of diarrhoea. On each occasion the stool contains segments of undigested vegetables. The paediatrician recommends restricting fluids to meal times. The girls condition improves and she is thriving.

268. A mother and her daughter have just returned from a tropical holiday and is concerned that her daughter has an STD, since she complains of constant perianal and vulval irritation. There is no associated vaginal discharge. She has worms coming out of her bottom at night.

269. A 15-year-girl complains of episodic diarrhoea which typically starts in the morning with a constant urge to

go to the toilet on waking, and after breakfast. She says there is associated abdominal pain in the right iliac fossa relieved by defaecation or flatus. She has had the symptoms for 3 months.

Theme Investigation of Possible Thromboembolic Disease

Options

A. Chest X-ray

B. Coagulation screen

C. Contrast spiral computed tomography (CT) scan

D. Digital subtraction angiography

E. Echocardiography

F. Femoral duplex scan

G. Magnetic resonance imaging (MRI) scan

H. Platelet count

I. Selective arteriogram

J. Ventilation perfusion scan

Instructions

For each patient described below,choose the *single* most likely discriminating investigation from the above list of options. Each option may be used once, more than once, or not at all.

270. A 29-year-old woman, who has been taking the oral combined pill for six months, is brought to the Accident and Emergency Department in a state of collapse. Her blood pressure is 70/40mmHg and she has raised neck veins.

271. A 23-year-old woman, who has been taking the oral combined pill for six months, presents with bilateral ankle oedema and a tender calf.

272. A 20-year-old woman, who has been taking the combined pill for six months presents with a history of cough, producing green sputum, and fever, over the last two or three days.

273. A 22-year-old woman, who has been taking the pill for six months presents with palpitations and on examination has a diastolic murmur and thrill.

Theme Management of Acute Chest Pain

Options

A. Glyceryl trinitrate (0.5mg) Sublingually

B. IV 50 ml of 50% dextrose

C. High flow O_2 and ramipril 2.5 mg/12hr PO

D. High flow O_2, 10mg iv morphine + anticoagulation

E. Cross match blood and inform surgeons

F. Insert a 16 G cannula in second intercostal space

G. IV heparin 5000-10,000 iu over 5 min

H. Underwater seal drainage

I. 10 mg IV diamorphine

J. Nifedine

Instructions

For each patient described below, choose the *single* most appropriate immediate measure to take from the above list of options. Each option may be used once, more than once or not at all.

274. A tall young woman developed sharp pain on one side of his chest two days ago. Since then he has been short of breath on exertion.

275. After a heavy bout of drinking a 56-year-old man vomits several times and develops chest pain. When you examine him, he has a crackling feeling under the skin around his neck.

276. A 23-year-old woman on the oral contraceptive pill suddenly gets tightness in her chest and becomes very breathless.

277. A 30-year-old man with Marfan's syndrome has sudden central chest pain going through to the back.

278. A 57-year-old man develops crushing pain in the chest associated with nausea and profuse sweating. The pain is still present when he arrives in hospital an hour later.

Theme Treatment of Oesophageal Pathology

Options

A. Endoscopic dilatation
B. Ketonazole systemically administered
C. Topical nystatin
D. IV ganciclovir
E. IV acyclovir (High dose)
F. IV acyclovir (Low dose)
G. Surgical resection
H. Endoscopic insertion of Atkinson tube
I. Heller's myotomy
J. Triple therapy
K. Surgical repair
L. Sclerotherapy

Instructions

For each of the patients described below, choose the most appropriate treatment from the options listed above. Each option may be used once, more than once, or not at all.

279. A 32-year-old man has been receiving cyclosporin for the treatment of her rheumatoid arthritis presents with odynophagia (painful swallowing) and mild dysphagia. Oesophageal endoscopy reveals multiple small white plaques on background of an abnormally reddened mucosa.

280. A 31-year-old woman with AIDS presents with odynophagia. Oesophageal endoscopy reveals multiple shallow ulcers in the lower oesophagus. The mucosa contains multiple vesicles.

281. A 29-year-obese man presents with dysphagia. Barium swallow demonstrates a smooth 'rat tail ' appearance. He has complained of heartburn for the last 6 months.

282. A 62-year-old woman presents with dysphagia. He says it's been progessive, having started with initial difficulty for swallowing solids, but now also now has involved liquids. He looks wasted.

Theme Investigations of Patient with Haemoptysis

Options

A. Computed tomography

B. Fibreoptic bronchoscopy

C. Fine needle aspiration

D. Mediastinoscopy

E. Mediastinotomy

F. Magnetic resonance imaging (MRI)

G. Pulmonary angiogram

H. Selective arteriogram

I. Sputum culture

J. Sputum cytology

K. Thoracoscopy

L. Ventilation perfusion scan

Instructions

For each suspected diagnosis below, choose the *single* most definitive investigation from the above list of options. Each option may be used once, more than once, or not at all.

283. Tuberculosis.
284. Carcinoma of the right main bronchus.
285. Pulmonary embolism
286. Bronchiectasis.
287. Bronchial carcinoid.

Theme Diagnosis of Complications of Cholecystectomy

Options

A. Acute pancreatitis

B. Acute renal failure

C. Biliary peritonitis

D. Inferior venacava thrombosis

E. Myocardial infarction

F. Pulmonary embolism

G. Small bowel obstruction

H. Stone in common bile duct

I. Sub-phrenic abscess

Instructions

For each test result below, choose the *single* most likely complication of cholecystectomy from the above list of options. Each option may be used once, more than once or not at all.

288. Chest X-ray shows raised right diaphram with small pleural effusion above.

289. Ultrasound scan shows intra-abdominal free fluid with paralytic ileus.

290. Liver function tests show raised alkaline phosphates, raised bilirubin, normal albumin and normal hepato-cellular enzymes.

291. Ultrasound scan shows dilated common bile duct with no free intra -abdominal fluid or bowel distension.

292. Chest X-ray shows signs of left ventricular dilatation and an electrocardiograph (ECG) shows Q waves with ST elevation.

Theme Diagnosis of Chest Pain

Options

A. Angina pectoris

B. Acute myocardial infarction

C. Bronchiectasis

D. Hiatus hernia

E. Pneumonia

F. Pulmonary embolism

G. Pleural effusion

H. Tension pneumothorax

I. Lung fibrosis

J. Reflux oesophagitis

K. Spontaneous pneumothorax

L. Aortic dissection

M. Possible malignant change

Instructions

For each patient described below, choose the *single* most likely diagnosis from the list of options above. Each option may be used once, more than once, or not at all.

293. A 70-year-old man has had malaise for five days and fever for two days. He has a cough and you find stony dullness, on percussion at the right lung base.

294. A 53-year-old woman returned by air to the UK from Washington. Three days later she presents with sharp chest pain and breathlessness. Her chest X-ray and ECG are normal.

295. A tall, thin 23-year-old man has a sudden pain in the chest and left shoulder and breathlessness while cycling.

296. A 49-year-old porter presents with a two hour history of chest pain radiating into the left arm. His ECG is normal.

297. A 52-year-old obese man has had episodic anterior chest pain, particularly at night, for three weeks. Chest X-ray and ECG are normal.

Theme Progression of Breast Cancer

Options

A. Asthma

B. Axillary recurrence

C. Bone marrow infiltration

D. Bony metastasis

E. Cerebral

F. Hypercalcemia

G. Left ventricular failure

H. Liver metastases

I. Local occurence

J. Lymphagitis carcinomatosis

K. Peritoneal recurrence

L. Pleural effusion

M. Spinal cord compression

Instructions

For each patient described below, choose the *single* most likely diagnosis from the above list of options. Each option may be used once, more than once, or not at all.

298. A 56-year-old woman who underwent mastectomy for a breast tumour four years ago, now complains of increasing breathlessness. On examination of her respiratoiy system, she is noted to have decreased movement of the left hemithorax which is dull to percussion and has absent breath sounds.

299. A 60-year-old woman is admitted to the Accident and Emergency Department having fallen in the street. She is complaining of pain in the right hip and the right lower limb is lying in external rotation. She had breast conserving surgery, radiotherapy and chemo-therapy eight years ago for breast cancer.

300. A 43-year-old woman treated two years ago for a Grade 3 axillary node positive breast cancer presents with increasing confusion, headache and vomiting. On examination, she is drowsy but has no focal neuro-logical signs. She does have blurring of the optic disc margins.

301. A 35-year-old woman treated one year ago for a breast cancer with 12/20 nodes positive, presents with a two day history of increasing confusion. She is drowsy and disorientated. Her husband reports that she has been complaining of severe thirst for the past week.

302. A 45-year-old woman treated three years ago for breast cancer is unable to walk. She complains of increasing weakness in her left leg for the last seven days. She has been constipated and unable to pass urine for the last 24 hours.

Theme Diagnosis of Acute Abdomen

Options

A. Acute pancreatitis
B. Acute cholecystitis
C. Acute myocardial infarction
D. Pyloric stenosis

E. Intestinal obstruction
F. Appendicular abscess
G. Acute appendicitis
H. Acute pyelonephritis
I. Possible ruptured ectopic
J. Aortic dissection
L. Possible twisted ovarian cyst
M. Oesophageal varices

Instructions

For each patient described below, choose the *single* most likely diagnosis from the list of options above. Each option may be used once, more than once or not at all.

303. A 74-year-old man with a previous history of pain in his calves in walkings, is brought to the Accident and Emergency Department, after having collapsed in the street. He is complaining of abdominal pain radiating to his back.

304. A 24-year-old woman presents to the Accident and Emergency Department with a sudden onset of left iliac fossa pain. She is pale and has a pulse of 120 beats/min with a BP of 105/65 mmHg. On examination of her abdomen she is tender in her left iliac fossa.

305. A 36-year-old woman presents with a 12 hour history of severe epigastric pain associated with several episodes of vomiting. She drinks about 40 units of alcohol per week. She is tender with guarding in the epigastrium. Plain radiography shows no evidence of free gas.

306. A 40-year-old man is admitted with a history of 24 hours of colicky central abdominal pain and bile stained vomiting. His only past medical history is an appendicectomy when he was 8. On examination his abdomen is distended, but there is no tenderness. Bowel sounds are increased.

307. A fit 18-year-old man presents with a 12 hour history of central abdominal pain radiating to his right iliac fossa. He is pyrexial with tenderness, guarding and rebound in the right iliac fossa.

Theme Causes of Pneumonia

Options

A. Aspiration

B. Bronchiectasis

C. Fungal

D. *Haemophilus influenzae*

E. Klebsiella

F. Lung cancer

G. Mycoplasma pneumonia

H. *Pneumocystitis carinii*

 I. *Staphylococcus aureus*

J. *Streptococcus pneumoniae*

K. Tuberculosis

L. Viral pneumonia

M. Legionella pneumophila

Instructions

For each patient described below, choose the *single* most likely underlying cause from the above list of options. Each option may be used once, more than once, or not at all.

308. A 35-year-old woman presents with a four month history of cough, productive o sputum, and recent haemoptysis. She has lost 5 kg in weight. The chest X-ray shows right upper lobe consolidation.

309. A previously well 18-year-old has had influenzae for the last two weeks. She is deteriorating and has a swinging fever. She is coughing up copious purulent sputum. Chest X-ray shows cavitating lesions.

310. A 65-year-old man, currently undergoing chemotherapy for chronic leukemia, has felt unwell with fever and an unproductive cough for two weeks despite treatment with broad spectrum intravenous antibiotics. The chest X-ray shows an enlarging right sided, mid-zone consolidation.

311. A 27-year-old male prostitute has felt generally unwell for two months with some weight loss. Over the last three weeks he has noticed a dry cough with increasing breathlessness. Two courses of antibiotics

from his GP has produced no improvement. The chest X-ray shows bilateral interstitial infiltrates.

312. On return to university, a 20-year-old student presented with the onset of fever, malaise and a dry cough. The student health service gave him amoxycillin. After a week he felt no better and his chest X-ray showed patchy bilateral consolidation.

313. A 64-year-old man with chronic obstructive pulmonary disease, presents with pneumonia. Clinically he improves with antibiotics. In the outpatient clinic four weeks later, the consolidation on his chest X-ray has not resolved.

314. A 27 year old male patient has just returned from holiday abroad presents with mild flu-like illness, headaches, high fever prior to this, he had complained of abdominal pain, vomiting, diarrhoea associated with blood per rectal.

Theme Treatment of Infectious Disease

Options

A. Ganciclovir

B. Pyrimethamine + Sulphadiazine

C. No treatment required

D. Bed rest and avoid alcohol

E. Interferon alpha

F. Co-trimoxazole

G. Zidovudine (AZT), Didanosine (ddi) + Ritonavir

H. Lamivudine, stavudine, + AZT

I. Fluconazole

J. Flucloxacillin

K. Ribavirin

L. Antihistamines and careful observation for one week

Instructions

For each of the patients described, choose the most appropriate treatment from the list of options above. Each option may be used once, more than once or not at all.

315. A 23-year-old male homosexual presents with tachycardia, tachypnoea and a dry cough, associated

with exertional dyspnoea. Chest X-ray shows a granular appearance. Echocardiography is normal.

316. A 20-year-old female air hostess presents to the dermatology clinic where she is found to have seborrheic dermatitis. On examination she is found to have oral candidiasis and dusky red lesions on the buccal mucosa. Further examination reveals axillary and supraclavicular lymphadenopathy. She has lost weight in recent months.

317. A 23-year-old woman presents with a mild dry cough and running nose. She is found to have enlarged axillary nodes and a maculo-papular rash all over the body which she says developed after taking ampicillin at home.

318. A 32-year-old known HIV patient presents with headache, photophobia. He is found to have a CD4 count of 99 cells/ml. A computed tomography scan shows ring enhancing lesions.

Theme Diagnosis of Thromboerobolism

Options

A. Inferior venacava obstruction
B. Superior Venacava obstruction
C. Lymphoedema
D. Deep vein thrombosis
E. Pneumonia
F. Bronchiectasis
G. Aortic stenosis
H. Mitral stenosis
I. Pulmonary embolism
J. Ruptured Baker's cyst
K. Venous insufficiency

Instructions

For each of the patients described below, choose the *single* most likely diagnosis from the list of options above.

319. A 26-year-old female security who has been taking the combined oral contraceptive pill for six months, presents with bilateral ankle oedema which has been

present for six months. There is no calf tenderness but the skin over her legs is itchy and pigmented.

320. A 31-year-old woman, who has been taking the oral contraceptive pill for six months, is brought to the Accident and Emergency Department in a state of collapse. Her blood pressure is 70/40mmHg and her neck veins are raised.

321. A 40-year-old woman who has complained of joint pain, stiffness and swelling that are worse in the morning for 5 years and is receiving steroids for her illness. She has been off the pill for one year, but now presents with a sudden onset severe right calf pain.

322. A 30-year-old woman, who has been taking the oral contraceptive pill for six months, presents with palpitations and on examination, a mid diastolic murmur is found.

323. A 23-year-old woman, who has been taking the combined oral contraceptive pill for six months, presents with a history of cough, producing green sputum, and fever, over the last two or three days.

Theme Antibiotic Prophylaxis of Surgical Patients

Options

A. Angiography
B. Bronchoscopy
C. Colle's fracture
D. Dental treatment of a cardiac patient
E. Dislocated shoulder
F. Emergency appendicectomy
G. Heart valve replacement
H. Sigmoid colectomy
I. Splenectomy
J. Thyroidectomy

Instructions

For each prophylactic regimen given below, choose the *single* most likely indication from the above list of options. Each option may be used once, more than once or not at all.

324. 3 gm sachet of amoxycillin one hour before the procedure.
325. Three days of intravenous broad spectrum antibiotics beginning with induction of anaesthesia.
326. Clear fluids by mouth and two sachets of sodium picosulphate on the day before the operation plus broad spectrum intravenous antibiotics at induction.
327. Long term oral penicillin and immunisation against pneumococcal infection.
328. One dose of metronidazole at induction of anaesthesia.

Theme Diagnosis of Headache

Options

A. Carotid artery stenosis
B. Cerebellar haemorrhage
C. Temporal neuralgia
D. Cerebral vasculitis
E. Migraine
F. Subarachnoid haemorrhage
G. Chronic subdural haematoma
H. Polymyalgia rheumatica
 I. Vertebro basilar TIA
 J. Temporal arteritis
K. Pagets disease
L. Cluster headache

Instructions

For each patient described, choose the *single* most likely diagnosis from the above list of options. Each option may be once, more than once or not at all.

329. A 42-year-old business man, has a history of headaches associated with photophobia and phonophobia- The headaches always follow a flight from Edinburgh were he has business interests.
330. A deaf 56-year-old woman complains of a chronic headache. She is found to have sabre tibiae.

331. A 59-year-old man previously in good health, presents with sudden onset of severe occipital headache and vomiting. Her only physical sign on examination is a stiff neck.

332. A 38-year-old woman suffers paroxysms of intense stabbing pain, lasting only a few seconds in the face. It's precipitated by talking.

333. A 34 years chronic alcoholic had a fall two weeks ago. He now presents with slowly increasing drowsiness and headache.

Theme the Management of Patients in a Coma

Options

A. Alcohol level

B. Angiography

C. Arterial blood gases

D. Blood cultures

E. Blood sugar

F. Computed tomography (CT)

G. Naloxone

H. Paracetamol screen

I. Plasma osmolality

J. Toxicology

K. Urea and electrolytes

Instructions

For each patient described below, choose the *single* most appropriate intervention from the options above. Each option may be used once, more than once, or not at all.

334. A 25-year-old found deeply unconscious is brought to the Accident and Emergency Department. He has an abrasion over his left temple and puncture marks on his left forearm.

335. A 37-year-old alcoholic is found wandering in a park. His partner says he has had a number of falls recently and in the Accident and Emergency the patient is confused. The blood sugar level is normal.

336. A 19-year-old university student went home from class because of a headache.The next morning she is found unconscious at home. She has a purpuric rash and a fever.

337. A 23-year-old known diabetic arrives in the Accident and Emergency Department. She is pale, sweaty and unconscious. Her companion says she was well 30 minutes ago, but suddenly became confused and then could not be roused.

338. A 45-year-old is brought to the Accident and Emergency Department by her husband who reports that she collapsed in the bathroom. Upon examination, she is unconscious with bilateral upgoing plantar responses. Her blood sugar level is normal.

Theme Prescribing for Pain Relief

Options

A. A bolus of intravenous opiate

B. A subcutaneous opiate infusion

C. Acupuncture

D. Carbamazepine

E. Corticosteroids

F. Hypnotherapy

G. Intramuscular non-steroidal anti-inflammatory drugs (NSAIDS)

H. Oral non-steroidal anti-inflammatory drugs (NSAID)

I. Oral opiates

J. Proton pump inhibitors (eg. omeprazole)

K. Selective serotonin re-uptake inhibitor eg. fluoxetine

L. Simple analgesics

M. Transcutaneous electrical nerve stimulation (TENS) machine

N. Tricyclic antidepressant

Instructions

For each patient dscribed below, choose the *single* most appropriate method of pain relief from the above list of options. Each option may be used once, more than once or not at all.

339. A 65-year-old man presents with severe, retrosternal chest pain and sweating. An ECG shows an acute infero-lateral myocardial infarction.

340. A 70-year-old man with inoperable gastric cancer causing obstruction, and multiple liver metastases, is taking a large dose of oral analgesia. Despite this, his pain is currently unrelieved.

341. A 25-year-old woman has just been diagnosed a havin rheumatoid arthritis and her rheumatologist has begun giving her gold injections. She continues to complain of joint pain and stiffness, particularly for the first two hours of each day.

342. A 50-year-old obese man with a known hiatus hernia, presents with recurrent, severe, burning retrosternal chest pain associated with acid regurgitation and increased oral flatulence.

343. A 67-year-old woman reports severe paroxysms of knife -like or electric shock-like pain, lasting seconds, in the lower part of the right side of her face.

344. A 27-year-old man presents with an 8-year history of back pain, worse in the morning, and one episode of uveitis.

Theme the Diagnosis of a Red Eye

Options

A. Acute glaucoma
B. Conjuctivitis
C. Dacryocystitis
D. Dacryoadenitis
E. Endopthalmitis
F. Foreign body
G. Scleritis
H. Spontaneous subconjuctival haemorrhage
I. Trachoma
J. Trauma
K. Uveitis

   L. Episcleritis
   M. Herpes zoster ulcer
   N. Dendritic ulcer
   O. Ulcerative keratitis

Instructions

For each patient described below, choose the *single* most appropriate diagnosis from the above list of options. Each option may be used once, more than once, or not at all.

345. A 60-year-old patient presented to his GP with sudden onset of redness in the left eye. There was no pain and the vision was unaffected.

346. A 72-year-old patient complains of severe pain in his right eye with severe deterioration of vision. He had noticed haloes around street lights for a few days before the onset of pain.

347. A seven-year-old North African boy gave a history of two years of discomfort, redness and mucopurulent discharge affecting both eyes. His two siblings have a similar problem.

348. A 24-year-old man has a history of recurrent attacks of blurring of vision associated with redness, pain and photophobia. Both eyes have been affected in the past. His older brother is currently being investigated for severe backache.

349. A 35-year-old rugby player sustained facial injuries. Twelve months later he presented with a painful swelling at the left medial canthus, associated with red eye and purulent discharge.

350. A 24-year-old man with a painful red eye, has his eye stained with fluorescein drops. Areas of the cornea are stained yellow. Steroid eye drops are given and massive ulceration and blindness results.

Theme Antepartum Haemorrhage-the Selection and Interpretation of

Options

   A. Biophysical profile (eg. foetal heart monitoring)
   B. Cord blood flow studies (Doppler)

C. Central venous pressure

D. Coagulation profile

E. Cardiotocography

F. Electronic maternal cardiovascular monitoring (ECG/Electrocardiogram)

G. Placental localisation (USS/Ultrasound scan)

H. Haemoglobin

I. Kleihauer test

J. Pulse oximetry

K. Rhesus status

L. Speculum examination

M. Urinalysis

Instructions

For each patient described below, choose the *single* most appropriate investigation from the above list of options. Each option may be used once, more than once or not at all.

351. A 24-year-old gravida 4 para 3, presents with a painless, unprovoked vaginal bleed of approximately 50 ml at 32 weeks. She is generally well, but worried.

352. A 25-year-old nullipara presents at 26 weeks gestation with slight postcoital bleeding.

353. Following recurrent antepartum haemorrhage, investigation shows the foetus to be small for dates at 32 weeks. Conservative management is preferred. A 19-week foetal anomaly ultrasound scan confirmed normal placental localisation.

354. A woman, whose previous pregnancy was complicated by iso-immunisation, has vaginal spotting at 36 weeks in an otherwise normal pregnancy.

355. A 31-year-old woman is anxious about slight per vaginal bleeding. She is 22 weeks pregnant and had similar complaints 2 years ago when she was on the pill.

Theme Ethical Practice of Medicine in the UK

Options

A. Tell the police

B. Don't tell the police

C. Ask the girl to come with parent/guardian, as procedure can't be carried out without their approval

D. Talk to girl about importance of telling parents but just
go on and cary out procedure if she refuses to tell
parents

E. Offer the contraception only with parental consent
only.

F. Offer contraception if risks are discussed, even without
parental consent

G. Consult with senior managers of the the NHS trust

H. Tell partner of the patient's illness

I. Don't tell partner since the patient is against this

J. Consult with social services

Instructions

For each of the scenarios described below, choose the most
appropriate action to be taken. Each option may be used
once, more than once or not at all.

356. A 13-year-old girl is pregnant and requires a termination of the pregnancy. She tells you emphatically that
at no point should you consider informing her
parents.

357. An armed robber is injured during an exchange of
gunfire with the police and comes to the Accident and
Emergency Department, and naturally requests your
silence.

358. A 13-year-old girl is having unprotected sex with her
17-year-old boy friend and asks that she be given the
oral contraceptive pill.

359. A 32-year-old man is found to be HIV positive. He is
against condom use and, after a lengthy talk with him
refuses to accept the need to tell his wife.

360. A 30-year-old man is pulled over while driving for
suspected drink driving. A breath test proves negative
and the patient says its probably the medication you
prescribed that is to blame. The police call you and
request that you tell them what medicine you
prescribed the man. The man then calls you and asks
that you don't tell the police.

Theme Prescribing for Alcohol and Drug Abuse

Options

A. Acamprosate

B. Admit and give benzodiazepines

C. Benzodiazepines

D. Disulfiram

E. Electroconvulsive therapy (ECT)

F. Haematinics

G. Heroin

H. High potency vitamins

 I. Insulin coma therapy

J. Lithium

K. Liver extract

L. Methadone

M. Multivitamins

N. Naltrexone

O. Refer to substance misuse team

P. Vitamin K

Instructions

For each patient described below, choose the *single* appropriate treatment from the above list of options. Each option may be used once, more than once or not at all.

361. A 46-year-old man presents to the clinic with a history of shakes for 12 hours, which started after he woke up following a 36 hour binge of alcohol at a party.

362. A 34-year-old unemployed man has been in hospital for a period of detoxification due to alcohol. He is ready for discharge but wants to remain abstinent after discharge.

363. A 27-year-old woman wants help in coming off heroin. She attends the Accident and Emergency Department. She has been injecting heroin intermittently for the last six months. Her partner is not a drug user and is very supportive.

364. A 46-year film maker presents with making up stories to fill the memory gaps. He shows global amnesia on

testing and there is no impairment of consciousness. He gives a history of alcohol abuse and has been hearing voices. He is already taking vitamin supplements.

365. A 46-year-old woman has been admitted to the medical ward with jaundice and a past history of alcohol abuse. She is now seeing ants crawling over her and is becoming disturbed and restless.

Theme Decision Making in Terminal Care

Options

A. Add amitriptyline or similar drugs
B. Add midazolam/methotrimeprazine
C. Antibiotics
D. Administer enema
E. Gastric intubation
F. High fibre diet
G. Increase opiate analgesia
H. Intravenous fluids
I. Nutritional supplements
J. Palliative deep X-ray therapy
K. Prescribe bisphosphates
L. Prescribe laxative
M. Reduce opiate analgesia
N. Set up syringe driver
O. Start steroids
P. Pleurodesis
Q. Intercostal nerve block
R. Betadine gel
S. High dose frusemide

Instructions

For each patient described below, choose the *single* most appropriate action from the above list of options. Each option may be used once, more than once, or not at all.

366. A 70-year-old woman with terminal endometrial carcinoma is distressed by a very foul vaginal discharge.

367. A 70-year-old woman with terminal breast carcinoma gets recurrent pleural effusions.

368. A 70-year-old woman with metastatic bowel carcinoma is distressed by severe pleural pain. She is already on 80 mg/12h PO of diamorphine.

369. An 80-year-old man with metastatic carcinoma becomes confused with abdominal distension and faecal incontinence. He is on high doses of opiates.

370. A 55-year-old woman with known spinal metastases from breast cancer becomes nauseated and confused. Creatinine is 120 mmol/L; blood sugar is 5.4 mmol/L; calcium 3.2 mmol/L. She is receiving intravenous fluids.

371. A 45-year-old man is dying of pain of AIDS (Acquired Immunodeficiency Syndrome). He is in considerable pain, despite the morphine sulphate, slow release, 20 mg daily; amitriptyline 100 mg at night and Naproxen 500mg twice a day.

372. A 65-year-old man with prostate cancer has extensive pelvic spread of disease with pain not adequately controlled by full analgesic cover.

373. An 82-year-old man with bronchial carcinoma is distressed by breathlessness. He is depressed and anorexic, but in no pain.

Theme Diagnosis of Acute Abdominal Pain in Younger Women

Options

A. Acute gastroenteritis

B. Acute pancreatitis

C. Appendicitis

D. Biliary colic

E. Cholecystitis

F. Ectopic pregnancy

G. Mesenteric thrombosis

H. Perforated peptic ulcer

I. Renal colic

J. Salpingitis

K. Spontaneous abortion

L. Strangulated hernia

M. Torsion ovarian cyst

N. Ulcerative colitis

O. Urinary tract infection (UTI)

Instructions

For each patient described below, choose the *single* most likely diagnosis from the above list of options. Each option may be used once, more than once or not at all.

374. A 20-year-old married woman presents in the Accident and Emergency Department with the onset of acute lower abdominal pain. Her last menstrual period was six weeks previously. She has pain radiating to the left shoulder.

375. A 15-year-old girl presents with a 24 hour history of central abdominal pain, followed by the right iliac fossa pain, worse on coughing. She has fever and rebound in the right iliac fossa.

376. A 30-year-old woman has severe colic and upper abdominal pain radiating to her right scapula and is vomiting.

377. A 12-year-old girl has central abdominal pain and is vomiting. On examination, her abdomen is found to be distended with no rebound and a tender lump in the right groin.

378. A 31-year-old woman has severe colic and upper abdominal pain. She is febrile and vomiting. Haematological investigations show a moderate leucocytosis.

379. A 31-year-old woman presents with acute, severe abdominal pain. Her blood pressure is 100/60mmHg and no abdominal signs are found. Haemoglobin level is 17g/dl and the plasma amylase is only mildly raised.

Theme Diagnosis of Menstrual Disorders (Amenorrhoea)

Options

A. Anorexia

B. Complete androgen insensitivity

C. Hyperthyroidism

D. Hypogonadal hypogonadism
E. Hypothyroidism
F. Intra-uterine synaechia
G. Menopause
H. Polycystic ovarian syndrome
I. Pregnancy
J. Premature ovarian failure
L. Prolactinoma
M. Turner's syndrome
N. Bulimia

Instructions

For each patient described below, choose the *single* most likely diagnosis from the above list of options. Each option may be used once, more than once, or not at all.

380. An 18-year-old dancer presents with secondary amenorrhoea. On examination, she is 1m 68 cm tall and weighs 46 kg.

381. A 34-year-old woman presents with an eight month history of secondary amennorrhea. On direct questioning she admits to a weight loss of 6 kg despite having a good appetite.

382. A 19-year-old woman presents with an eight month history of secondary amenorrhoea. Prior to this her periods have been irregular since the menarche at the age of 12. Her body mass index (BMI) is 32.

383. A 33-year-old woman presents with a seven month history of amenorhoea. She also complains of hot flushes, night sweats and mood swings.

384. A 17-year-old girl with secondary amenorrhoea, is reported to be binge eating. She has a BMI of 16 is concerned that she is fat and goes to the gym 4 times a day, on all days of the week.

Theme Immediate Management of an Injured Patient

Options

A. Abdominal ultrasound
B. Assess airway

C. Cervical spine immobilisation

D. Chest auscultation

E. Chest drain after needle thoracocentesis

F. Computed tomography (CT) brain scan

G. Electrocardiogram (ECG)

H. Endotracheal intubation

I. Immediate blood transfusion

J. Rapid (20 min) fluid bolus (1 litre)

K. Splint femoral fracture

L. Transfer to operating theatre

M. X-ray femur

Instructions

For each patient described below, choose the *single* most likely immediate action from the above list options. Each option may be used once, more than once, or not at all.

385. A 22-year-old motorcyclist, in the Accident and Emergency Department resuscitation room, appears to be stable after an accident. While sitting up talking, he becomes progessively breathless. There is reduced air entry on the left side of his chest.

386. A 22-year-old motorist arrives in the Accident and Emergency Department after an accident. His airway is patent. He is noted to have external injuries on the left side and a deformed left thigh.

387. A 22-year-old motorist is being resuscitated after an accident. His airway is secure.Pulse rate is 110 beats/min, blood pressure 100/50 mmHg, Glasgow Coma Scale 9. He has a deformed left thigh.

Theme Premaligant Malignant Disease

Options

A. Erythoplasia of querat

B. Marjolins ulcer

C. Malignant melanoma

D. Pytriasis versicolor

E. Dermatofibroma

F. Lentigo maligna

G. Basal cell carcinoma

H. Porokeratosis

I. Squamous cell carcinoma

J. Solar keratosis

K. Pyogenic granuloma

L. Lupus vulgaris

M. Psoriasis

N. Seborrhoeic keratosis

O. Bowen's disease

Instructions

For each of the patients described below, choose the **single** most approprite answer from the list of options above. Each option may be used once, more than once or not at all.

388. A 56-year-old man who works in Australia for most of the year presents with cutaneous scaling on his arms and forehead. There is no history of progression, induration and no obvious ulceration is seen on examination.

389. A retired 55-year-old man who worked in an arsenic factory presents with a flat scaly, red crusted plaque on his right hand. He says it's progessively increased in size.

390. A 45-year-old woman presents with multiple marked brown lesions on the fore head and limbs.

391. A 36-year-old woman presents with multiple scaly lesions on the upper trunk and back, which seem to disappear and recur.

392. A 56-year-old man presents with a shallow ulcerative lesion on the right cheek. It has pearly rolled margins.

393. A 65-year-old uncircumcised man is found to a red scaly lesion on his penis. The consultant dermatologist confirms, it's bowen's disease.

Theme Mechanism of Poisoning

Options

A. Aspirin

B. Ipratopium

C. Paracetamol

D. Cyanide

E. Steroids

F. Quinine

G. Carbon monoxide

H. Oxygen

I. Morphine

J. Warfarin

K. Heparin

L. Cocaine

M. Amphetamine

N. Glue

Instructions

For each of the conditions below, choose the single most appropriate action to take. Each option may be used once, more than once or not at all.

394. When would you use acetylcysteine as an antidote?

395. When would you use methionine as an antidote?

396. What can cause heart block?

397. Sodium nititrite followed by sodium thiosulphate would be useful.

398. Protamine sulphate is used in overdosage with it.

399. Dicobalt edetate is a useful antidote.

400. Methadone is useful for those who are addicted.

Theme Investigation of Aortic Aneurysms

Options

A. Computed tomography

B. Ultrasound of abdomen

C. ECG

D. Echocardiography

E. Ankle-femoral index

F. Coronary angiogarphy

G. Doppler ultrasound

H. Intravenous pyelography

I. Spiral computed tomography

J. Immediate surgery

K. IV normal saline

L. O negative blood transfusion

M. Chest X-ray

Instructions

For each of the patients described below, choose the *single* most appropriate investigation, from the list of options above. Each option may be used once, more than once or not at all.

401. A 68-year-old man with an aortic aneurysm is being considered for surgery. In addition he has had a myocardial infarction and intermittent claudication.

402. A 68-year-old woman with an aortic aneurysm is being considered for surgery. You are assesing for renal involvement.

403. A 68-year-old man presents with a pulsatile mass in the abdomen.

404. A 68-year-old man with an abdominal aortic aneurysm presents with calf tenderness and a positive Homan's sign.

405. A 68-year-old man with an abdominal aortic aneurysm presents with sudden onset epigastric pain. His blood pressure is 60/40 mmHg and pulse rate is 200 beats/min.

Theme Diagnosis of Dysphagia

Options

A. Achalasia

B. Benign stricture

C. Pharyngeal pouch

D. Carcinoma of the oesophagus

E. Oesophagitis

F. Peptic stricture

G. Myasthenia gravis

H. Plummer-Vinson syndrome

I. Globus hystericus

J. Diffuse oesophageal spasm

K. Oesophageal candidiasis

L. Mallory-Weiss syndrome

M. Schatzki ring

Instructions.

For each of the patients below, choose the *single* most likely diagnosis from the list of options above. Each option may be used once, more than once or not at all.

406. A 43-year-old woman complains of difficulty in swallowing both liquids and solids. He is found to have a red tongue and angular stomatitis.

407. A 45-year-old man had a renal transplant 6 months ago. He now complains of painful swallowing.

408. A 34-year-old man presents with a history of intermittent dysphagia of both liquids and solids. He gets temporary relief on eating large quantities of food. There is a further history nocturnal retrosternal chest pain but he denies any loss in weight.

409. A 59-year-old man complains of progessive difficulty swallowing solids. In the last 2 days he has noticed a difficulty in swallowing liquids and says anorexia has made him lose weight.

410. An obese 45-year-old man complains of difficulty in swallowing. In addition he complains of retrosternal chest pain especially following heavy meals. He smokes about 25 cigarettes a day.

Theme Developmental Milestones

Options

A. 2-3 months

B. 0-2 months

C. 2-5 months

D. 7-10 months

E. 6-10 months

F. 10-13 months

G. 4-7 months

H. 15-18 months

I. 2-3 years

J. 11-14 months

K. 2-4 years

L. 6-8 years

Instructions

For each of the milestones below, choose the *single* most likely answer from the list of options above. Each option may be used once, more than once or not at all.

411. Smiles spontaneously.
412. Listen to bells.
413. Squeals.
414. Says 'Dada and Mama'
415. Sits alone.
416. Finger thumb grasp.
417. Drinks from cup.
418. Walks alone.
419. Pulls self to stand.
420. Walks around furniture.

Theme Antibiotic Prophylaxis of Surgical Patients

Options

A. Angiography

B. Bronchoscopy

C. Colles' fracture

D. Dental treatment of a cardiac patient

E. Dislocated shoulder

F. Emergency appendicectomy

G. Heart valve replacement

H. Sigmoid colectomy

I. Splenectomy

J. Thyroidectomy

Instructions

For each prophylactic regimen given below, choose the *single* most likely indication from the above list of options. Each option may be used once, more than once or not at all.

421. 3 g sachet of amoxycillin one hour before procedure.
422. Three days of intravenous broad spectrum antibiotics beginning with induction of anaesthesia.
423. Clear fluids by mouth and two sachets of sodium picosulphate on the day before the operation plus broad spectrum intravenous antibiotics at induction.
424. Long term oral penicillin and immunisation against pneumococcal infection.
425. One dose of metronidazole at induction of anaesthesia.

Theme Interpretation of Haematology Results

Options

A. Alcoholism
B. Beta thalassaemia major
C. Chronic blood loss
D. Cytotoxic drugs
E. Dietary deficiency
F. Haemolysis
G. Hypothyroidism
H. Pernicious anaemia
I. Rheumatoid arthritis
J. Untreated hyperthyroidism

Instructions

For each set of results below, choose the *single* most likely cause from the above list of options. Each option may be used once, more than once, or not at all.

426.	Hb	7.9g/dL
	MCV	57fL
	MCHC	21g/dL
	WBC	$9.0 \times 1,000,000,000$/L
	Platelets	$523 \times 1,000,000,000$/L
	Retics	6%
	ESR	14 mm/hr
427.	Hb	10.9g/dL
	MCV	106fL
	MCHC	37g/dL
	WBC	$8.0 \times 1,000,000,000$/L
	Platelets	$223 \times 1000,000,000$/L

	Retics	< 1%
	ESR	8 min/hr
	Blood film	Target cells
428.	Hb	5.6g/dL
	MCV	83fL
	MCHC	32g/dL
	WBC	1.3 × 1,000,000,000/L
	Platelets	62 × 1,000,000,000/L
	Retics	< 1%
	ESR	6 min/hr
	Blood film	Normal
429.	Hb	9.8g/dL
	MCV	84fL
	MCHC	33g/dL
	WBC	7.1 × 1,000,000,000/L
	Platelets	194 × 1,000,000,000/L
	Retics	< 1%
	ESR	90 min/hr
	Blood film	Normal
430.	Hb	10.1g/dL
	MCV	73fL
	MCHC	31g/dL
	WBC	6.1 × 1,000,000,000/L
	Platelets	283 × 1,000,000,000/L
	Retics	9%
	ESR	15 min/hr
	Blood film	Small irregular shaped RBC, anisocytosis

Theme Diagnostic Test for Patients Presenting with Chest Pain

Options

A. Abdominal ultrasound

B. Blood culture

C. Bronchoscopy

D. Cardiac enzymes

E. Chest X-ray

F. Computed tomography (CT)

G. Electrocardiogram (ECG)

H. Full blood count (FBC)

I. Lumbar puncture

J. Oesophago-gastro-duodenoscopy

K. Ventilation/Perfusion scan

Instructions

For each patient described below, choose the *single* next most appropriate test from the above list of options. Each option may be used once, more than once, or not at all.

431. A 68-year-old man has had malaise for five days and fever for two days. He has a cough and you find dullness to percussion at the left lung base.

432. A 50-year-old woman returned by air to the UK from Australia. Three days later she presents with sharp chest pain and breathlessness. Her chest X-ray and ECG are normal.

433. A tall, thin, young man has a sudden pain in the chest and left shoulder and breathlessness while cycling.

434. A 45-year-old manual worker presents with a two hour history of chest pain radiating into the left arm. His ECG is normal.

435. A 52-year-old obese man has had episodic anterior chest pain, particularly at night, for three weeks. Chest X-ray and ECG are normal.

Theme Risk Factors of Opthalmic Pathology

Options

A. Myopia

B. Hypermetropia

C. Astigmatism

D. Hereditary in 30%

E. Hypocalcemia

F. Polycythaemia rubra vera

G. Immunosuppression

H. Candidiasis

I. Myxoedema

J. Sjogren's syndrome

Instructions

For each patient described below with opthalmic disease, choose the *single* most likely risk factor from the list above

436. A 38-year-old man suddenly notices markedly reduced vision in his right eye. He cannot read the visual acuity chart and can only count fingers. The fundus looks red and intensely hypaeremic.

437. A 57-year-old man complains of sudden loss of vision in his right eye. She describes the incident like 'a curtain coming down'.

438. A 59-year-old man says he is always running into objects.His vision is blurred and also complains of dazzling in bright light.

439. A 39-year-old woman complains of a gritty feeling in her eyes. A schirmers test is performed and is found to be positive.

Theme the Immediate Management of Meningitis

Options

A. Acyclovir

B. Antipyretics

C. Cranial computed tomography (CT) scan

D. High dose steroids

E. Intravenous (IV) 20% dextrose

F. Intravenous (IV) plasma expansion

G. Intravenous (IV) sodium bicarbonate

H. Lumbar puncture

I. Naso-gastric tube insertion

J. Thick and thin blood film

K. Treat immediate contacts

L. Urinary catheter

Instructions

For each patient described below, choose the *single* most urgent first step from the above list of options. Each option may be used once, more than once, or not at all.

440. A four-year-old girl, who has never been immunised, has been treated with ampicillin for otitis media. After five days she is more unwell with fever, headache, photophobia, neck stifiness but no alteration in consciousness. Her fundi and blood pressure are normal.

441. A previously well college student aged 18, is found unconscious by his friend. On arrival at the Accident and Emergency Department, he has a tachycardia, weak pulse and a rapidly spreading purpuric rash. His college doctor has given him intramuscular penicillin.

442. A 23-year-old unemployed woman who is known to have AIDS has a three week history of increasing vomiting, headache and weight loss. On examination she is confused and has papilloedema and brady-cardia.

443. A six-week-old boy developed fever, neck stifiness and photophobia on the morning after his birthday. He has a petechial rash and antibiotics were started for suspected meningococcal infection. He is now stable and receiving all necessary immediate treatment.

444. A 40-year-old journalist visited Western Africa at short notice for three days.24 hours after returning home, he has sudden fever, rigor and stiff neck and shoulders. On examination he has excoriated urticarial lesions of his ankles and mild jaundice.

Theme Ethical Practice of Medicine

Options

A. Resuscitate without consent and do cervical smear since this may be only opportunity

B. Resuscitate even without consent

C. Wait for relatives before you can begin resuscitation

D. Transfuse with blood

E. Don't transfuse with blood, even if patients' life is at risk

F. Inform relevant health authority

G. Respect the patient's confidentiality, don't inform health authority

H. Respect the patient's confidentiality and don't tell lawyer

I. Tell lawyer about her condition without her consent

J. Ask for consent again

K. No need to ask for consent again

Instructions

For each of the scenarios below choose the most appropriate action to take from the above list of options. Each option may be used once, more than once or not at all.

445. A 17-year-old boy is brought into the Accident and Emergency Department unconscious, following a road traffic accident.

446. You are treating a surgeon for Hepatitis B, you ask him to inform the NHS trust where he is working and he refuses.

447. A 32-year-old woman is brought into the Accident and Emergency Department, by her husband drifting in and out consciousness, following a road traffic accident. She is in shock and you decide she needs an immediate blood transfusion. Her husband objects saying they are devout Jehovars' witnesses and are against blood transfusion. Her condition is deteriorating.

448. A 50-year-old wealthy widow has terminal breast cancer and has only days to live. She has confided in you before that her daughters are threatening to kill each other, over who inherits her estate and her enormous wealth. She has no will and her lawyer requests that you tell him whether her condition is terminal so he can convince her to sign the will. Informing her, about her worsening condition has caused significant deterioration in her condition before.

449. You are treating a 56-year-old woman who had an acute myocardial infarction. Her condition is not improving and you want your medical secretary to type a referral letter .The secretary asks for the patients' medical records so that she can type the letter.

Theme Investigation of Urinary Tract Infection (UTI)

Options

A. Abdominal X-ray

B. Intravenous urogram

C. Isotope renal scan

D. Laparotomy

E. Lumbosacral spine X-ray

F. Micturating cysto-urethrogram

G. Mid stream specimen of urine

H. Serum creatinine

I. Supra pubic aspiration of urine for culture

J. Urinary glucose test

K. Urodynamics

Instructions

For each child described below, choose the *single* most helpful next investigation from the above list of options. Each option may be used once, more than once, or not at all.

450. A 10 day old girl has developed fever and jaundice and is not feeding as well as normal. A bag urine specimen showed red and white cells and a culture of mixed organisms. Abdominal examination is normal.

451. A one-year-old boy had a severe urine infection complicated by *E. coli* septicaemia one month ago. Urine is now sterile. He is on prophylactic antibiotics. Utrasound examination of the abdomen during the acute infection was normal.

452. A five-year-old boy has a persistent history of diurnal and nocturnal enuresis and soiling. Abdominal examination is normal. A proteus urinary tract infection (UTI) has been confirmed on culture. He has had a series of orthopaedic operations for talipes equino varus.

453. An eight-year-old girl presents with a 12 hour history of nausea and central abdominal pain now radiating to the right iliac fossa. She has urinary frequency.

454. A 14-year-old girl has had a pseudomonas urinary tract infection and her blood pressure is 140/95 mmHg persistently. She has a past history of recurrent urinary tract infections and an abdominal ultrasound at the age of two was normal.

Theme the Natural History of Joint Disease

Options

A. Ankylosing spondylitis
B. Gout
C. Osteoarthritis of the hip
D. Prolapsed intervertebral disc
E. Painful arc syndrome
F. Rheumatoid arthritis
G. Rotator cuff tear
H. Sjogren's syndrome
I. Systemic lupus erythromatosus
J. Tennis elbow
K. Tendinitis of long head of biceps
L. Psoriatic arthritis

Instructions

For each description below, choose the *single* most likely condition from the above list of options. Each option may be used once, more than once or not at all.

455. A condition which affects males more than females, which starts with inflammatory joint symptoms in late teens or early twenties. There is a gradual improvement in symptoms in later life.

456. A progressive, symmetrical, inflammatory arthritis with a relapsing and remitting course over several years resulting in significant destruction of several joints.

457. An acute presentation of back pain radiating down the leg with resolution in the majority of cases over a six week period. It may recover even without treatment.

458. Intermittent acute attacks of severe asymmetrical monoarthritis over a period of several years with symptom free intervals.

459. Shoulder pain which is only present between 45 and 160 degrees of abduction.

460. Pain is felt in the anterior shoulder and is characteristically worse on forced contraction of the biceps.

Theme the Diagnosis of Vaginal Bleeding

Options

A. Cervical carcinoma

B. Vulval carcinoma

C. Cervical ectropion

D. Endometrial carcinoma

E. Endometriosis

F. Ectopic pregnancy

G. Ovarian carcinoma

H. Menopause

I. Hyperthyroidism

J. Rhesus incompatibility

K. Von willebrand's disease

L. Pelvic infammatory disease

M. Pelvic adhesions

Instructions

For each patient described below, choose the *single* most likely diagnosis from the options listed above. Each option may be used once, more than once or not at all.

461. A 50-year-old woman presents with a nine month history of prolonged, slightly irregular periods. Clinical examination shows a normal size uterus with no adnexal masses.

462. A 31-year-old nulliparous woman with a history of cyclical pelvic pain, complains of heavy and frequent periods. On vaginal examination a fixed retroverted uterus is found.

463. A 53-year-old woman has had a history of offensive vaginal discharge and intermittent vaginal bleeding over the past three months. Her husband died of carcinoma of the penis.

464. A 46-year-old woman who has breast cancer and is on tamoxifen has had two episodes of bright red bleeding. Her last period was when she started tamoxifen two years ago.

465. A 22-year-old woman with a six week history of amenorrhoea presents to the Accident and Emergency Department with vaginal bleeding. An ultrasound scan reports "an empty uterus."

466. An obese 55-year-old woman presents with per vaginal bleeding associated with a watery non-foul discharge. She is nulliparous. Her mother and father died of carcinoma colon.

Theme the Disease Process of Asthma

Options

A. 5% reversibility in FEV$_1$

B. 10% reversibility in FEV$_1$

C. 15% reversibility in FEV$_1$

D. Alpha receptors

E. Beta 2 receptors

F. Eosinophils

G. Forced vital capacity

H. Histamine

I. IgA

J. IgE

K. IgG

L. IgM

M. Leukotrienes

N. Mast cells

O. Neutrophils

P. Peak expiratory flow rate (PEFR)

Q. Positive pollen skin test

R. Raised eosinophil count

S. T cells

T. Vital capacity

Instructions

For each of the statements below, choose the *single* most likely connecting statement from the above list of options. Each option may be used once, more than once, or not at all.

467. A criterion for the diagnosis of asthma.

468. The substance is released by mast cell activation and causes bronchospasm.

469. This parameter of respiratory function is usually unaffected by asthma.

470. Found commonly in the sputum of patients with asthma.

471. Blocking these can cause worsening of asthma.

Theme Clinical Management of Hypertension in Pregnancy

Options

A. 24 hour urinary protein

B. A period of observation for blood pressure

C. Complete neurological examination

D. Foetal ultrasound

E. Immediate ceasarean section

F. Induction of labour

G. Intravenous antihypertensives

H. Intravenous benzodiazepines

I. Low dose aspirin

J. Magnesium hydroxide

K. Oral antihypertensive

L. Oral diuretic

M. Recheck blood pressure in seven days

N. Renal function tests

O. Retinoscopy

Instructions

For each patient described below, choose the *single* most appropriate action from the above list of options. Each option may be used once, more than once, or not at all.

472. A patient in her third pregnancy presents to her GP at 12 weeks gestation. She was mildly hypertensive in both of her previous pregnancies. Her BP is 150/100 mmHg. Two weeks later, at the hospital ante-natal clinic, her BP is 150/95 mmHg.

473. A 24-year-old Nigerian woman has an uneventful first pregnancy to 30 weeks. She is then admitted as an emergency with epigastric pain. During the first 2 hours her BP rises from 150/105 mmHg to 170/120 mmHg. On dipstick she is found to have 3+ proteinuria. The foetal cardiogram (CTG) is normal.

474. At ante-natal clinic visit at 38 weeks gestation, a 36-year-old multiparous woman has a BP of 140/90 mmHg. She has no proteinuria, but she is found to have oedema to her knees.

475. At 32 weeks, a 22-year-old primigravida is found to have a BP of 145/100 mmHg. At her first visit at 12 weeks the BP was 145/90 mmHg. She has no proteinuria, but she is found to have oedema to her knees.

476. At 34 weeks, an 85 kg woman complains of persistent headaches and 'flashing lights'. There is no hyper-reflexia and her BP is 150/100 mmHg. Urinalysis is negative but she has finger oedema.

Theme Prescribing and Renal Failure

Options

A. Aluminium hydroxide

B. Aspirin

C. Bendrofluazide

D. Calcitriol

E. Calcium

F. Captopril

G. Diamorphine

H. Enalapril

I. Frusemide

J. Insulin -increased dosage

K. Insulin-reduced dosage

L. Magnesium

M. Mefenamic acid

N. Metoprolol

O. Metformin

P. Paracetamol

Q. Spironolactone

Instructions

For each patient described below, choose the *single* most appropriate drug to prescribe from the above list of options. Each option may be used once, more than once, or not at all.

477. A 30-year-old man with diabetes mellitus and severe renal failure (serum creatinine 700 umol/l - x 7 normal) has a blood glucose concentration of 24 mmol/L (x 3 normal).

478. A 43-year-old woman with severe renal failure (serum creatinine concentration 750 umol/l -x 7.5 normal) presents with markedly swollen ankles.

479. A 21-year-old man with a failing renal transplant (serum creatinine concentration 600 umol/l - x 6 normal) has a blood pressure of 220/142 mmHg).

480. A 62-year-old man with chronic renal failure (serum creatinine concentration 800 umol/l - x 8 normal) and known renal calculi presents with left sided renal colic.

481. A 20-year-old man with severe renal failure (serum creatinine 700 umol/l presents with proximal myopathy.

Theme Prescribing and liver failure

Options

A. Spironolactone 100 mg/24hrPO

B. Frusemide 100 mg/24hr PO

C. Paracentesis

D. Paracentesis with albumin infusion

E. Ciprofloxacin 250 mg PO

F. Flucloxacillin 500 mg/24hr PO

G. Chloropheniramine 75 mg PO

H. Cholestyramine 4g/8hPO

I. Tetracycline 250 mg/8h PO

J. Stop warfarin

K. Warfarin-increased dosage

L. Warfarin-reduced dosage

M. Bed rest, salt and fluid restriction

Instructions

For each patient described below choose the most appropriate drug/action from the above list of options.

482. A 32-year-old chronic alcoholic is in liver failure.He has severe pruritus.

483. A 30-year-old chronic alcoholic is on warfarin following an acute myocardial infarction, he suffered 3 months ago. He now develops liver cirrhosis.

484. A 32-year-old man has had hepatitis B for the last one year and now presents with a grossly distended abdomen and other stigmata of liver disease. You are worried he may develop spontaneous bacterial peritonitis.

485. A 30-year-old woman presents with a mildly distended abdomen, yellowing of the mucous membranes. She is found to have spider naevi on her chest.

Theme Staging and Prognosis

Options

A. 90%

B. 65%

C. 30%

D. 20%

E. 70%

F. 80%

G. 5%

H. 10%

I. 100%

Instructions

For each of the patients with cancer described below, match the appropriate stage with the expected 5-year survival treatment if adequate treatment is given. Each option may be used once, more than once or not at all.

486. A 59-year-old man presents with bleeding per rectum. He is found to have colorectal carcinoma confined to the bowel wall.

487. A 79-year-old man with a history of weight loss and per rectal bleeding is found to large bowel carcinoma with paraortic lymph node involvement.

488. A 71-year-old woman with tenesmus and bleeding per rectum has bowel carcinoma which has not involved any lymph nodes but has penetrated the bowel wall.

489. A 55-year-old woman with a foul smelling vaginal discharge and post-coital is found to have stage II cervical carcinoma.

490. A 40-year-old woman presents with a 3 month history of postal coital bleeding. She is found to have stage I cancer of the cervix.

Theme Association of
Systemic Disease and Skin Lesions

Options

A. Erythema chronicum migrans

B. Erythema multiforme

C. Pretibial myxoedema

D. Dermatitis herpetiformis

E. Livedo (a cutaneous vasculitis)

F. Dermatomyositis

G. Bazins disease

H. Dermatitis artefacta

I. Alopecia areata

L. Mycosis fungoides

M. Bowen's disease

N. Paget's disease

O. Rodent ulcer

P. Cafe au lait spots

Instructions

For each of the diseases named below, choose the most likely matching skin pathology from the list of options above. Each option may be used once, more than once or not at all.

491. Addison's disease
492. Cutaneous T-cell lymphoma
493. Coeliac disease
494. Hyperthyroidism
495. Tuberculosis
496. Polyarteritis nodosa
497. Mycoplasma pneumoniae
498. Lyme disease
499. Von Recklinghausen's disease
500. Bronchial carcinoma

Theme Headache: Selection of Diagnostic Tests

Options

A. Carotid arteriography

B. Computed tomography (CT) scan of the brain

C. Electroencephalogram (EEG)

D. Erythrocyte sedimentation rate (ESR)

E. Fundoscopy

F. Intraocular pressure

G. Lumbar puncture

H. Magnetic resonance imaging (MRI) of cervical spine

I. Mental state examination

J. Nasendoscopy

K. Skull X-ray

L. Temporal artery biopsy

M. Toxoplasma serology

N. Visual fields

Instructions

For each patient described below, choose the **single** most appropriate investigation from the above list of options. Each option may be used once, more than once or not at all.

501. A 30-year-old woman has a generalised headache, described as a tight band, unrelieved by paracetamol. She has difficulty in sleeping and has lost weight recently.

502. A 54-year-old man has a severe headache, worse on lying. You find bilateral papilloedema.

503. A 68-year-old woman has a right sided headache aggravated by brushing her hair. She says she has been generally unwell for a few months with aching muscles.

504. A 13-year-old boy presents with drowsiness and generalised headache. He is recovering from a bilateral parotitis. His CT scan is normal.

505. A 30-year-old man presents with headache, photophobia and sudden reduction in visual acuity. His fundi look pale.

506. A 34-year-old known HIV positive South African man presents with a generalised headache. Computed tomography is done and shows ring enhancing lesions.

Theme Incubation Periods for Common Diseases

Options

A. 15-50 days

B. 50-180 days

C. 10-20 years

D. 7-21 days

E. 3 hours - 5 days

F. 9-90 days

G. 14-21 days

H. 20-40 years
 I. 3 days
 J. 60 days
 K. 5 hours
 L. 7-8 days
M. 11-21 days

Instructions

For each of the disease conditions listed below choose the most appropriate incubation period from the list of options above. Each option may be used once, more than once or not at all.

507. Measles
508. Chicken pox
509. Rubella
510. Mumps
511. Hepatitis B
512. Hepatitis A
513. Cholera
514. Syphilis
515. Creutzfeldt-Jakob's disease (CJD)

Theme the Management of Chronic Joint Pain

Options

A. Allopurinol

B. Antidepressant

C. Cognitive behavioural therapy

D. Colchicine

E. Gold

F. Joint replacement

G. Methotrexate

H. Oral non-steroidal anti-inflammatory drugs (NSAID)

 I. Oral non-steroidal anti-inflammatory drugs (NSAID) with gastric protection

J. Joint aspiration and blood culture

K. Paracetamol

L. Sulphasalazine

Instructions

For each patient described below, choose the *single* most likely initial management from the above list of options. Each option may be used once, more than once, or not at all.

516. A 50-year-old obese asthmatic businessman who, drinks 40 units of alcohol a week, presents with fifth episode of a red hot ankle. Aspiration of the joint has revealed uric acid crystals.

517. A healthy 70-year-old independent woman complains of increasing pain in her left knee and episodes of the joint 'giving way'. She is no longer able to climb her stairs. On examination, she is found to have a marked valgus deformity with obvious instability.

518. A 43-year-old woman with long-standing rheumatoid arthritis, presents with a red, swollen, inflamed right knee. She has a swinging pyrexia.

519. A 20-year-old brick layer with ankylosing spondylitis has increasing early morning back pain and stiffness. He is on no medication at present.

520. An elderly man with severe ischaemic heart disease complains of stiff, painful hands, neck, knees and feet. Examination of the hands reveals Herberden's nodes.

Theme Diagnosis of Personality Disorders

Options

A. Histrionic personality disorder
B. Borderline personality disorder
C. Schizotypal personality disorder
D. Schizoid personality disorder
E. Panic attack disorder
F. Paranoid personality disorder
G. Obsessive-compulsive personality disorder
H. Avoidant personality disorder
 I. Antisocial personality disorder
J. Dependent personality disorder

Instructions

For each patient described below choose the *single* most likely diagnosis from the list of options above. Each option may be used once, more than once or not at all.

521. A 20-year-old man keeps cleaning his hands every time he shakes his partner's hands. He was a high achiever in high school.

522. A 56-year-old farmer believes his 34-year-old neighbour is killing his farm animals despite the local veterinary's advice that the death is due to an outbreak of anthrax. He spends hours watching his neighbour through pair of binocular lens, hoping to catch in the act.

523. A 16-year-old girl is described as 'queer' by his mates. She is unfriendly and has no close friends despite numerous attempts by boys in her college. She lacks empathy and is largely introspective.

524. A 16-year-old girl in high school always comes late to class wearing strong perfume in a vain attempt to attract attention. She laughs loudly at jokes, many of her mates don't find particularly hilarious.

525. A 32-year-old man always gives in to his wife over any decision even when he knows this isn't right. He insists on having his wife prepare his every meal, wash him and put him to sleep. He cries whenever his wife's away.

Theme the Management of Joint Pain

Options

A. Allopurinol
B. Carbamazepine
C. Hypnosis
D. Colchicine
E. Penicillamine
F. Prothesis consideration
G. Methotrexate
H. Ibuprofen
I. Naproxen with gastric protection

J. Joint aspiration and blood culture

K. Paracetamol

L. Sulphalazine

M. Acupuncture

N. Drain and await culture results

O. Drain and start on 250 mg flucloxacillin 6 hrly

Instructions

For each patient described below, choose the *single* most likely initial management from the above list of options. Each option may be used once, more than once or not at all.

526. A 43-year-old man has had a chronic knee joint pain for 3 years. He has been given loads of medication and requests alternative treatment. He dislikes surgery, as his brother died during an appendicectomy.

527. A healthy 80-year-old independent woman complains of creasing pain in her left knee and episodes of the joint 'giving way '. She is no longer able to walk her dog. She is found to have a marked valgus deformity with obvious instability and muscle wasting.

528. A 30-year-old woman with long-standing rheumatoid arthritis, presents with a red, swollen, inflamed right knee. She a swinging pyrexia, associated with rigors.

529. A 19-year-old student with ankylosing spondylitis has increasing early morning back pain and stiffness. He is on no medication at present.

530. An elderly woman with multiple sclerosis complains of stiff, painfull hands, neck, knees and feet. Examination reveals bouchards' nodes on the hands.

531. A 6-year-old girl is unwilling to show her right hand which is swollen, tender and warm. She is pyrexial.

Theme: Treatment of Depression

Options

A. Electroconvulsive therapy

B. Flupenthixol

C. Psychodynamic psychotherapy

D. Conginitive therapy

E. Behavioural therapy

F. Marital therapy

G. Lithium

H. Imipramine

I. No action

J. Psychosurgery

K. Hypnotherapy

L. Abreaction

M. Counselling

Instructions

For each patient described below, choose the *single* most appropriate treatment from the list of options. Each option may be used once, more than once or not at all.

532. A 15-year-old girl with a BMI of 16 complains of a 6 week history of ammenorhoea. She is not on the pill and her pregnancy test is negative. She wants to be a model.

533. A 20-year-old woman presents with inability to sleep and aggressiveness and increased libido. Her husband says prior to this she was markedly withdrawn and blamed herself for their daughter's death due leukemia. She feels life is not worth living.

534. A 14-year-old boy refuses to go to school because of constant failure to score grade A. He is threatening to drown himself.

535. A 20-year-old first time mother presents a week after delivering with episodes of crying and feeling alone.

536. A 40-year-old man has been treated for depression for 5 months. He has lost several kgs in weight and is getting suicidal thoughts.

Theme the Management of Red Eye

Options

A. No treatment

B. Check blood pressure and do coagulation studies

C. Immediate antibiotic therapy

D. Enucleation

E. 0.5% Prednisolone drops 4hrly

F. 0.5% Prednisolone drops 2hrly and cyclopentolate drops

G. 3% Pilocarpine drops and acetazolamide

H. 500 mg acetazolamide

I. Acyclovir drops

J. Total iridectomy 15 % flourescein drops

Instructions

For each patient described below, choose the *single* most appropriate mode of management from the above list of options. Each option may be used once more than once or not at all.

537. A 69-year-old patient presented to his GP with sudden onset of redness in the right eye. There was no pain and vision was unaffected.

538. A 60-year-old patient complains of severe pain in his left eye with severe deterioration of vision. He had noticed haloes around street lights at night for a few days before the onset of the pain.

539. A mother brings her 2-year-old child with a squint. On examination a leucokoric right pupil is seen with an absent red reflex.

540. A 12-year-old Libyan boy gave a two week history of discomfort, redness and mucopurulent discharge affecting both eyes. His two siblings have a similar problem.

541. A 23-year-old man has a history of recurrent attacks of blurring of vision associated with redness, pain and photophobia. Both eyes have been affected in the past. His older is currently being investigated for bowel disease and a severe backache.

542. A 25-year-old cricket player sustained facial injuries. 10 months later he presented with a painful swelling at the left medial canthus, associated with red eye and purulent discharge.

Theme Diagnosis of Dementia

Options

A. Alcoholic dementia

B. Alzheimer's dementia

C. Creutzfeldt-Jakob's disease

D. Head trauma

E. Human immunodeficiency virus (HIV)

F. Huntingtons chorea

G. Parkinsonism

H. Pick's disease

I. Repeated trauma

J. Space occupying lesions

K. Substance induced dementia

L. Toxin dementia

M. Vascular dementia

Instructions

For each patient described below, choose the *single* most likely diagnosis from the above list of options. Each option may be used once more than once or not at all.

543. A 50-year-old man with no previous history is brought to the Accident and Emergency Department by his wife who says that he has become progressively more forgetful, tends to lose his temper and is emotionally labile. There is no history of infectious disease or trauma.

544. A 74-year-old, man presents with weakness in his arm and leg (from which he recovered within a few days) and short term memory loss. He has an extensor plantar response. He had a similar episode two years ago and became unable to identify objects and to make proper judgements.

545. A 30-year-old sickler from Nigeria who received several blood transfusions a few years ago presents with irritability and increasing memory deficit. He is unable to speak properly. He is on pneumocystis carinni treatment.

546. A 39-year-old woman presents with memory loss, poor concentration and inability to recognise house hold objects. On examination she has right handed involuntary writhing movement. There is a strong family history of similar complaints.

547. A 69-year-old patient with chronic schizophrenia presents with a mask like face and involuntary pill rolling movement in both hands. He complains of chronic cough and forgetfullness.

Theme Management of Thromboembolic Disease

Options

A. Phlegm microscopy, culture and sensitivity

B. Echocardiography

C. Blood culture

D. Blood transfusion

E. Duplex scan

F. IV bolus of warfarin

G. 20 mg aspirin 12hrly

H. Coronary angiography

I. Counselling

J. Streptokinase

K. Protamine sulphate

L. Diathermy

M. Positron emission tomography (PET)

N. Cervical smear

O. Abdominal ultrasound

P. Dilatation and curettage

Instructions

For each patient described below, choose the *single* most important first management step from the above list of options. Each option may be used once, more than once, or not at all.

548. A 30-year-old woman, who has been taking the combined oral contraceptive pill for 9 months, is brought to the Accident and Emergency in a state of collapse. Her blood pressure is low and has a loud P2 on auscultation.

549. A 31-year-old woman is being treated for a thrombophilic tendency. The nurse administers dose of subcutaneeous Heparin and she begins to bleed from the nose and other injection sites.

550. A 26-year-old obese woman, presents with palpitations. On examination she is febrile and has nail bed fluctuance. He had previously presented with a diastolic murmur of mitral stenosis.

551. A 25-year-old woman, who has been taking the combined oral contraceptive pill for 2 months, presents with a 3 month history of cough with sputum, fever and night sweats. Her partner died of road traffiic accident.

552. A 16-year-old woman, who has been taking the pill for six months, presents with complaints of bleeding every month in her pill free days. Her mother died of cervical carcinoma.

Theme Diagnosis of Complications of Abdominal Surgery

Options

A. Mesenteric adenitis
B. Pulmonary embolism
C. Biliary peritonitis
D. Acute mesenteric thrombosis
E. Sub-phrenic abscess
F. Cholestasis
G. Small bowel obstruction
H. Posterior myocardial infarction
 I. Splenic rupture
J. Deep vein thrombosis
K. Wound dehiscence
L. Incisional hernia
M. Antero-lateral myocardial infarction
N. Inferior myocardial infarction

Instructions

For each patient below, choose the *single* most likely complication of abdominal surgery from the above list of options. Each option may be used once, more than once or not at all

553. Ultrasound shows intra-abdominal free fluid.
554. Blood pressure is 80/60 mmHg and pulse rate is 110 bts/min.
555. ECG shows Q waves and ST elevation in leads III and VF

556. Liver function tests show raised alkaline phosphates, raised bilirubin, normal albumin and normal hepato-cellular enzymes.

557. 5 days following cholecystectomy, incision wound is noted to have a serous discharge.

558. Days following bowel resection, a 45-year-old man presented with chest pain on inspiration and haemoptysis. JVP is raised and the P2 is loud on auscultation.

Theme Investigations of Patient with a Productive Cough

Options

A. Computed tomography (CT) scan
B. Ziehl nielsen (ZN) staining
C. Echocardiography
D. Ventilation perfusion scan
E. Broncho-pulmonary lavage
F. Sputum cytology
G. Mediastinoscopy
H. Mediastinostomy
I. Pulmonary angiography
J. Thoracoscopy
K. Selective arteriogram
L. Magnetic resonance imaging (MRI) scan
M. Fibre optic bronchoscopy

Instructions

For each suspected diagnosis below, choose the *single* most definitive investigation from the above list of options. Each option may be used once, more than once, or not at all.

559. Pnuemocystis carinii pneumonia
560. Tuberculosis
561. Bronchial carcinoma
562. Bronchiectasis
563. Bronchial carcinoid
564. Pulmonary embolism

Theme Immediate Management of a Trauma Patient

Options

A. Plain abdominal X-ray

B. Asses airway and stabilize spine

C. CT scan of abdomen

D. Transfer to operating theatre

E. Call ambulance only after full recovery

F. Chest drain after needle thoracentesis

G. Electrocardiogram

H. Immediate blood transfusion

I. Cervical spine immobilisation

J. Bolus of 50% dextrose followed by a saline infusion

K. Computed tomography (CT) brain scan

L. Normal saline infusion

M. Burr hole(s) should drilled

N. Lumbar puncture

O. Call neuro-surgeon immediately

P. Splint limb

Instructions

For each patient described below choose the *single* most likely immediate action from the above options. Each option may be used once, more than once, or not at all.

565. A 43-year-old man is brought to the Accident and Emergency Department delirious, following and injury at a rugby match.His Glasgow Coma Scale (GCS) at the scene of injury is 13. On examination, his right pupil is fixed and dilated and GCS is now 7. Initial resuscitation has been done. The neuro-surgeon is 30 minutes away.

566. A 22-year-old motorist arrives in the Accident and Emergency Department after an accident. His airway is patent. He is noted to have a splinted right leg.

567. A 30-year-old man is involved in a fight. He has a bruise on the cheek. He complains of an acute abdominal pain and is vomiting. He had a herniorraphy

two weeks ago. He is conscious and fundoscopy hasn't been done.

568. A 29-year-old motorist, in the Accident and Emergency Department resuscitation room, appears to be stable after an accident. While standing up, he becomes progessively dyspnoeic. There is reduced air entry on the left side of his chest.

569. An 18-year-old girl is being resuscitated after an accident. Her airway is secure. She complains of neck pain.Her pulse rate is 100 beats/min and blood pressure is 110/70 mmHg. Glagsow Coma Scale is 13. She has a deformed left thigh.

570. A 22-year-old motorist is being resuscitated after an accident. He is noted to have external injuries on the right side and a deformed right hand.

Theme Causes of Pneumonia

Options

A. Legionella pneumophila
B. Tuberculosis
C. Fungal
D. *Haemophilus influenzae*
E. Bronchial carcinoma
F. *Mycoplasma pneumoniae*
G. *Pneumocystis carinii*
H. *Staphylococcus aureus*
I. Viral pneumonia
J. *Streptococcus pneumoniae*
K. Bronchiectasis
L. Klebsiella
M. Aspiration pneumonia

Instructions

For each patient described below, choose the *single* most likely underlying cause from the above list of options. Each option may be used once, more than once or not at all.

571. A 34-year-old male patient has just returned from Thailand. He presents with a mild flu like illness,

headaches, high fever. Prior to this, he had presented with per rectal bleeding, abdominal pain, diarrhoea and vomiting.

572. A 30-year-old man presents with a 3 month history of a productive cough. He has lost considerable weight and has recently developed haemoptysis. Chest X-ray shows left lower lobe consolidation.

573. A 26-year-old woman has had influenza for the last 2 weeks. She is not improving and has a swinging fever. She is coughing up copious amounts of purulent sputum. Chest X-ray shows cavities in both upper zones.

574. A 70-year-old man, currently on steroid treatment for ulcerative colitis, has felt unwell with fever and a dry cough for two weeks despite treatment with IV broad-spectrum antibiotics. The chest X-ray shows an enlarging, right sided, mid zone consolidation.

575. A 34-year-old haemophiliac, has felt generally unwell for two months with some weight loss. Over the last three weeks he has noticed a dry cough with increasing breathlessness. Two courses of antibiotics from his GP has produced no improvement. The chest X-ray shows bilateral interstial infiltrates.

576. On return to university, a 23-year-old student presented with onset of fever, malaise an dry cough. The student health service gave him amoxycillin. After a week he felt no better and his chest X-ray showed patchy bilateral consolidation.

577. A 60-year-old man with chronic obstructive pulmonary disease, presents with pneumonia. Clinically he improves with antibiotics. In the out patient clinic 5 weeks later the consolidation on his chest X-ray has not resolved.

578. A 32-year-old woman is rushed to theatre for an emergency appendectomy. During induction of general anaesthesia, she throws up.

Theme Diagnosis of Acute Abdominal Pain and Vomiting in Children

Options

A. Hirchsprungs disease

B. Pyloric stenosis

C. Acute cholecystitis

D. Duodenal atresia

E. Intussusception

F. Wilm's nephroblastoma

G. Mesenteric thrombosis

H. Gastro-oesophageal reflux

I. Meningitis

J. Meconium ileus

K. Cyclical vomiting

L. Necrotizing enterocolitis

M. Psychogenic vomiting

N. Urinary tract infection

O. Acute pancreatitis

P. Gastroenteritis

Instructions

For each child described below, choose the **single** most likely diagnosis from the above list of options. Each option may be used once, more than once, or not at all.

579. A 5-month-old baby presents with vomiting, following a 2 hour history of abdominal pain associated with drawing up of legs. The mother says her baby has passed reddish stool.

580. A 12-year-old girl presents with fever, flank pain. An abdominal mass is found on examination. Urine microscopy shows no haematuria.

581. An eight-year-old girl shows signs of moderate dehydration. She has vomited all fluids for 24 hours and the vomit is not bile stained. Her abdomen is now soft and non -tender. She has had two similar episodes in the past year.

582. A six-week-old breast fed girl had projectile vomiting after every feed for the past two weeks. She is now lethargic, dehydrated and tachypnoeic.

583. A one day old breast fed infant is vomiting after each feed. Abdominal X-ray demonstrated a "double bubble".

584. A 6-year-old febrile girl is drowsy and vomiting. She is being treated for otitis media by her GP.

585. 8 days after a premature birth, a mother notices her baby is crying excessively and has passed blood and mucus per rectal. The infant is still in the special care baby unit (SCBU)

586. A 15-year-old boy who is thriving has a mild abdominal pain and is passing "rice water" stools. She had been at a mates' birthday party the night before.

Theme Important Side Effects of Common Drugs

Options

A. Impotence
B. Wasting
C. Deep vein thrombosis
D. Bronchospasm
E. Pseudomembranous colitis
F. Haemorrhagic cystitis
G. Constipation
H. Retrobulbar neuritis
I. Endometrial carcinoma
J. Steven-Johnson syndrome
K. Retroperitoneal fibrosis

Instructions

For each of the drugs below, choose the *single* most important side-effect from the list of options above. Each option may be used once, more than once, or not at all.

587. Cimetidine
588. Cyclophosphamide
589. Diamorphine
590. Amoxycillin
591. Oral contraceptive pill
592. Aspirin
593. Ethambutol
594. Tamoxifen
595. Methysergide

Theme Diagnosis of Acute Chest Pain

Options

A. Acute pancreatitis
B. Angina pectoris
C. Aortic dissection
D. Trigeminal neuralgia
E. Herpes zoster
F. Lobar pneumonia
G. Ruptured oesophagus
H. Herpes simplex
 I. Acute myocardial infarction
J. Spontaneous pneumothorax
K. Acute cholecystitis
L. Bornholm disease
M. Tietze's syndrome
N. Oesophageal spasm
O. Fracture rib

Instructions

For each patient below, choose the *single* most likely diagnosis from the above list of options. Each option may be used once, more than once, or not at all.

596. A 23-year-old man develops pain an acute pain in her right chest radiating to her right shoulder associated with a fever. She is vomiting and has mild yellowing of her skin.

597. A tall young man developed sharp chest pain on his right, following a road traffic accident. On palpation, this area is tender. A chest X-ray shows her lungs are not injured.

598. A 23-year-old male prostitute develops severe chest pain. The area of chest pain corresponds to an area with an erythematous rash.

599. A 68-year-old man develops crushing chest pain in the chest associated with nausea and profuse sweating radiating to the neck. By the time he gets to hospital quarter of an hour later the pain is gone.

600. Minutes after upper GI endoscopy a 56-year-old man develops chest pain. When you examine him, he has a

crackling feeling under the skin around his upper chest and neck.

Theme Diagnosis of Common Infectious Diseases

Options

A. Measles
B. Tuberculosis
C. Meningitis
D. Sickle cell trait
E. Hepatitis A
F. Hepatitis B
G. Malaria
H. Acquired immune deficiency syndrome
I. Influenzae
J. Glandular fever
K. Chickenpox
L. Scarlet fever
M. Mumps
N. Rubella

Instructions

For each of the patients described below, choose the *single* most likely diagnosis from the list of options above. Each option may be used once more than once or not at all.

601. A 34-year-old man has lost 4 kg over the past 3 months, and complains of a 4 month history of a productive cough.

602. A 30-year-old man who has just returned from. Africa, complains of joint pains and fever associated with chills and rigors. A blood smear shows numerous 'ring' trophozoites.

603. A 23-year-old male homosexual complains of joint pains associated with malaise and mild icterus.

604. A mother brings her 2-year-old son to the Accident and Emergency Department, who is drowsy and vomiting. On examination, koplik spots were found with a generalised maculo-papular rash.

605. A 5-year-old girl was given antibiotics for an ear infection 6hrs ago, but is now afraid to look at bright light and has refuses to eat

Theme the Immediate Management of Meningitis

Options

A. Acyclovir

B. Antipyretics

C. Cranial computed tomography (CT) scan

D. High dose steroids

E. Intravenous (IV) 20% dextrose

F. Intravenous (IV) plasma expansion

G. Intravenous (IV) sodium bicarbonate

H. Lumbar puncture

I. Naso-gastric tube insertion

J. Thick and thin blood film

K. Treat immediate contacts

L. Urinary catheter

Instructions

For each patient described below, choose the *single* most urgent first step from the above list of options. Each option may be used once, more than once or not at all.

606. A six-year-old girl, who has never been immunised, has been treated with amoxycillin for otitis media. After five-days, she is more unwell with fever, headache, photophobia, neck stiffness but no alteration in consciousness. Her fundi and blood pressure are normal.

607. A previously welll college student aged 19, is found unconscious by his friend. On arrival at the Accident and Emergency Department, he has a tachycardia, weak pulse and a rapidly spreading purpuric rash. His college doctor has given him intramuscular penicillin.

608. A 32-year-old known AIDS patient has a three week history of increasing vomiting, headache and weight loss. On examination, she is confused and has papilloedema and pulse rate of 60 beats/min.

609. A seven-year-old boy developed fever, neck stiffness and photophobia on the morning after a schoolmates' birthday party. He has a petechial rash and antibiotics were started for suspected meningococcal infection. He is now stable and receiving all necessary immediate treatment.

610. A 43-year-old journalist visited Sierra Leone in west Africa to cover the on going war for 5 days. A day after returning at home in Islington, he has a sudden fever, rigors and stiff neck and shoulders. On examination he has excoriated urticarial lesions of his ankles and mild jaundice.

Theme Decision Making in the Injured Patient

Options

A. 10 units of soluble insulin (IV)

B. Secure airway and stabilize cervical spine

C. IV dexamethasone

D. 2 mg glucagon (IV)

E. Discharge patient after a period of counselling

F. 0.9% Saline (IV)

G. Splint limb

H. Asses airway

I. Aspirin

J. Morphine

K. Naproxen

L. 50 ml of 50% dextrose (IV)

M. Finger prick glucose measurement

N. Cut down should be performed

Instructions

For each of the scenarios below, choose the *single* most appropriate first step from the above list of options. Each option may be used once, more than once or not at all.

611. An obese 56-year-old man is involved in a road traffic accident and sustains multiple bruises. He now complains of severe excruciating pain in his right big toe. He had complained of a similar pain last year.

612. You arrive at the scene of major accident and find a 32-year-old man unconscious. He smells of alcohol.

613. A 34-year-old known diabetic is brought to the Accident and Emergency Department unconscious following a road traffic accident. Initial resuscitation has been done by the paramedics.

614. As part of the ambulance team you arrive at the scene of a major accident. You find a 19-year-old man unconscious smelling of alcohol. His airway and cervical spine are secured by your team.

615. After a heavy bout of drinking a 17-year-old is to the Accident and Emergency unconscious. The airway and cervical spine are secure. Several attempts at getting intravenous (iv) access have failed.

Theme the Natural History of Joint Disease

Options

A. Ankylosing spondylitis

B. Gout

C. Osteoarthritis of the hip

D. Prolasped intervetebral disc

E. Psoriatic arthritis

F. Rheumatoid arthritis

G. Sjogren's syndrome

H. Systemic lupus erythromatosus

I. Tennis elbow

J. Painful are syndrome

Instructions

For each patient described below, choose the *single* most likely condition from the above list of options. Each option may be used once more than once, or not at all.

616. A condition which affects males more than females, which starts with inflammatory symptoms in late

teens or early twenties. There is a gradual worsening of symptoms in later life.

617. A progressive, symmetrical, inflammatory arthritis with a relapsing and remitting course over several years resulting in significant destruction of several joints.

618. An acute presentation of back pain radiating down the leg with resolution in the majority of cases over a six-week period. It may recover even without treatment.

619. Intermittent acute attacks of a severe asymmetrical monoarthritis over a period of several years with symptom free intervals.

620. Shoulder pain which is present between 45 and 160 degrees of abduction.

Theme Prescription and Disease

Options

A. Vancomycin

B. Benzyl penicillin

C. Erythromycin

D. Actinomycin

E. Metronidazole

F. Amoxycillin

G. Glyceryl trinitrate (GTN)

H. Co-trimoxazole

I. Zidovudine (AZT)

J. Ondansetron

K. Fluconazole

L. Imidazole

M. Verapamil

N. Intravenous immunoglobulins (under senior guidance)

O. Piperacillin

P. Trimethoprim

Instructions

For each of the disease conditions mentioned below, choose the drug of choice from the above list of possible options. Each option may be used once, more than once or not at all.

621. *Meningococcal meningitis*
622. Tetanus
623. *Trichomonas vaginalis*
624. Vincent's angina
625. Uncomplicated urinary tract infection (UTI)
626. Pseudomembranous colitis (Patient allergic to vanco-mycin)
627. Sinusitis in patient allergic to penicillin
628. Acute otitis media
629. Acute streptococcal sore throat (patient allergic to penicillin)
630. *Pneumocystis carinii*
631. Amoebiasis

Theme the Management of Menopausal Symptoms

Options

A. Transdermal oestrogen patch

B. Raloxifene

C. Oestrogen implants

D. Oestrogen pessaries

E. Thyroid function tests

F. Vaginal lubricant

G. Regular exercise

H. Prophylactic hormone replacement therapy

I. Endometrial sampling

J. Cervical inspection

K. Cervical smear

M. High protein diet

Instructions

For each scenario below, choose the *single* most appropriate treatment from the above list of options. Each option may be used once, more than once or not at all.

632. A 34-year-old woman is worried about the menopause and wants advice on how best to reduce the incidence of osteoporosis

633. An obese 59-year-old post-menopausal woman presents with a two week history of per vaginal bleeding, which is becoming more frequent. She had previously been on tamoxifen.

634. An obese 40-year-old woman presents with a two history of post coital bleeding associated with a foul smelling vaginal discharge.

635. An obese 50-year-old pre-menopausal woman presents with menorrhagia. She complains of constipation and says, she can't stand cold weather.

636. A 56-year-old woman complains of night sweats and mood swings. She had a fracture neck of femur which is being treated. She denied a history of hot flushes. She has a family history of breast and endometrial carcinoma. She wants relief from her symptoms.

637. A 53-year-old who has a family history of breast cancer has been experiencing mild discomfort for a few hours following intercourse for the last month. She is worried about using hormones.

Theme Differential Diagnosis of Abdominal Pain in a Woman

Options

A. Uterine rupture

B. Ulcerative colitis

C. Twisted ovarian mass

D. Threatened miscarriage

E. Irritable Bowel Syndrome

F. Pelvic inflammatory disease

G. Renal colic

H. Endometriosis

 I. Appendicitis

 J. Acute pancreatitis

K. Ectopic pregnancy

L. Septic abortion

M. Break-through bleeding

N. Inevitable miscarriage

O. Missed abortion

P. Bowel carcinoma

Instructions

For each patient described below, choose the *single* most likely diagnosis from the above list of options. Each option may be used once, more than once or not at all.

638. A 35-year-old woman complains of abdominal discomfort relieved by passing flatus or defaecation. Over the last 6-month she has had episodes of diarrhoea and constipation, but denied she had lost weight. Her mother died of bowel carcinoma.

639. A 31-year-old man reports a 7-week history of gradual onset rectal bleeding associated with constipation. On examination he is found to have red eyes and skin lesions on both his shins. His brother had similar bowel symptoms and back pain.

640. A 17-year-old woman presents with a sudden onset of severe left iliac fossa pain. On vaginal ultrasound examination, 2cm echogenic masses are seen in the broad ligament. She says this pain seems to come on every month.

641. A 22-year-old has just had an Intra uterine device fitted. She complains of a watery brown, vaginal discharge and abdominal pain.

642. A 19-year-old woman presents as an emergency with a 3 hour history of lower abdominal pain and bleeding per vaginum. She has not seen her period for 8 weeks and had a positive home pregnancy test yesterday. On examination, the uterus is tender and bulky. The cervical os is closed.

643. A 32-year-old who conscientiously uses the oral contraceptive pill, has experienced monthly vaginal bleeding. On abdominal examination she is uncomfortable. Her temperature is 37°C, and is otherwise healthy.

Theme the Disease Process of Asthma

Options

A. 5% reversibility in FEV_1

B. 10% reversibility in FEV_1

C. 15% reversibility in FEV$_1$
D. Alpha receptors
E. Beta 2 receptors
F. Eosinophils
G. Forced vital capacity
H. Histamine
I. IgA
J. IgE
K. IgG
L. Spacer
M. Mast cells
N. Neutrophils
O. Peak expiratory flow rate (PEFR)
P. Captopril
Q. Raised eosinophil count
R. T cells
S. Vital capacity
T. Leukotrienes
U. Metre dose inhaler
V. Syringe driver
W. Positive pollen skin test
X. Aspirin

Instructions

For each of the statements below, choose the *single* most likely connecting statement from the above list of options. Each option may be used once more than once or not at all.

644. A device which aids the delivery of asthma medication in infants and young children.
645. Propanolol activation of these, is harzadous in asthma.
646. Immunoglobulins predominantly involved in atopic disease.
647. A criterion for the diagnosis of asthma.
648. Found commonly in the sputum of patients with asthma.
649. Medication contraindicated in asthmatics.
650. The substance is released on degranulation of mast cells and causes bronchospasm.
651. This parameter of respiratory function is usually affected by asthma.

652. This parameter of respiratory function is usually unaffected by asthma.
653. Important for the home monitoring of asthma control.

Theme Clinical Management of Hypertension in Pregnancy

Options

A. Low dose aspirin
B. A period of observation for blood pressure
C. 24 hour urinary protein
D. Foetal ultrasound
E. Retinoscope
F. Induction of labour
G. Renal function tests
H. Intravenous antihypertensive
I. Intravenous benzodiazepine
J. Magnesium hydoxide
K. Oral anti hypertensive
L. Oral diuretic
M. Recheck blood pressure in seven days
N. Complete neurological exam
O. Immediate caeserean section

Instructions

For each patient described below, choose the *single* most appropriate action from the above list of options. Each option may be used once, more than once or not at all.

654. A patient in her third pregnancy presents to her GP at 12-weeks gestation. She was mildly hypertensive in both of her previous pregnancies. Her BP is 150/100 mmHg. Two weeks later at the hospital antenatal clinic her BP is 150/95 mmHg

655. A 22-year-old Nigerian woman has an uneventful first pregnancy to 30 weeks. She is then admitted as an emergency with epigastric pain. During the first 2 hours her BP rises from 150/105 to 170/120 mmHg. On dipstick she is found to have 3+ proteinuria. The foetal cardiotocogram (CTG) is normal.

656. At an antenatal clinic visit at 38-weeks gestation, a 36-year-old multiparous woman has a BP of 140/90 mmHg. She has no proteinuria, and is otherwise well.

657. At 32 weeks, a 22-year-old primigravida is found to have a BP of 145/100 mmHg. She has no proteinuria, but she is found to have oedema to her knees.

658. At 34 weeks, a 86 kg woman complains of persistent headaches and 'flashing lights'. There is no hyper-reflexia and her BP is 150/100 mmHg. Urinalysis is negative but she has finger oedema.

Theme Headache: Selection of Diagnosis Tests

Options

A. Carotid arteriography
B. Computed tomography (CT) scan
C. Electroencephalogram (EEG)
D. Erythrocyte sedimentation rate (ESR)
E. Fundoscopy
F. Intraocular pressure
G. Lumbar puncture
H. Magnetic resonance imaging (MRI)
I. Mental state examination
J. Nasendoscopy
K. Skull X-ray
L. Temporal artery biopsy
M. Toxoplasma serology
N. Visual fields
O. Psychiatric history

Instructions

For each patient described below, choose the *single* most appropriate investigation from the above list of options. Each option may be used once, more than once, or not at all.

659. A 34-year-old woman has a generalised headache, described as a tight band, unrelieved by paracetamol. She has difficulty sleeping and says she has lost weight recently.

660. A 51-year-old man has a severe headache, worse on lying. You find bilateral papilloedema.

661. A 71-year-old woman has a severe headache aggravated by brushing her hair. She says she has been generally unwell for a few months with aching muscles.

662. A 14-year-old boy presents with drowsiness and generalised headache. He is recovering from a bilateral parotitis. His CT scan is normal.

663. A 32-year-old man presents with headache, photophobia and sudden reduction in visual acuity. His fundi look pale.

664. A 54-year-old man is brought to the Accident and Emergency with a 6-month history of headache. His wife says that he has also become progessively more forgetful, tends to lose his temper and is emotionally labile. There is no history of loss of weight, infectious disease or trauma.

665. A 55-year-old man with blurred vision complains of headache which he has had for the past 5 months. Coughing and sneezing seem to worsen the headache.

666. An obese 31-year-old woman is brought to the Accident and Emergency Department with a severe occipital headache of 2 hour duration. She is unable to move her left hand and leg.

667. A 23-year-old homosexual man complains of a headache of 3 week duration. A computed tomography scan is done and shows multiple 'ring' enhancing lesions.

668. A 34-year-old man with blurred vision complains of a severe headache of 1 hour duration. He also complains of pain on chewing.

Theme Drugs of Choice

Options

A. Diamorphine (IV)
B. Diamorphine (IM)
C. Salbutamol nebulised in oxygen
D. Nebulised steroids
E. Protamine sulphate
F. Carbamazepine
G. Donepezil
H. Methadone
I. Naltrexone

J. Vigabatrin

K. Sulphasalazine

L. Carbimazole

M. Carbamazepine

N. Propanolol

O. Radioiodine

P. Ipratopium bromide

Q. Diazepam

R. Paracetamol

S. Oxygen if needed and advice on risk factors

T. Fluoxetine

Instructions

For each patient described below, choose the *single* most appropriate drug from the above list of options. Each option may be used once, more than once or not at all. Each option may be used once, more than once or not at all.

669. A 65-year-old man with no previous history is brought to the Accident and Emergency Department by his wife who says that he has become progessively incontinent and forgetful and tends to have mood swings.

670. A 32-year-old 13-week pregnant woman complains of heat intolerance. She has lost weight despite a good appetite.

671. A 45-year-old man develops a crushing chest pain associated with nausea and profuse sweating. The pain is still present when he arrives in hospital an hour later.

672. A 13-year-old known asthmatic is brought to the Accident and Emergency Department breathless. Her pulse rate is 56 beats/min. No wheezing is heard.

673. A 32-year-old man has been treated for morphine dependence. He wants to stay off the drug.

674. The treatment of ulcerative colitis.

675. The treatment of crohn's disease.

676. A 45-year old man complains of morning stiffness of both his knees. On examination they are found to be swollen and tender. He has lost weight.

677. A 32-year-old man has lost weight since the death of his wife 3 months. He is withdrawn and has a bleak view of the future.

Theme Investigation of Urinary Tract Infection (UTI)

Options

A. Abdominal X-ray
B. Intravenous urogram
C. Isotope renal scan
D. Laparotomy
E. Lumbosacral spine X-ray
F. Micturating cysto-urethrogram
G. Mid–stream specimen of urine
H. Serum creatinine
I. Supra pubic aspiration of urine for culture
J. Urinary glucose test
K. Urodynamics

Instructions

For each child described below, choose the *single* most helpful next investigation from the above list of options. Each option may be used once, more than once, or not at all.

678. A 10 day old girl has developed fever and jaundice and is not feeding as well as normal. A bag of urine specimen showed red and white cells and a culture of mixed organisms. Abdominal examination is normal.

679. A one-year-old boy had a severe urine infection complicated by *E. coli* septicemia one month ago. Urine is now sterile. He is on prophylactic antibiotics. Ultrasound examination of the abdomen during the acute infection was normal.

680. A five-year-old boy has a persistent history of diurnal and nocturnal enuresis and soiling. Abdominal examination is normal. A proteus urinary tract infection (UTI) has been confirmed on culture. He has had a series of orthopaedic operations for talipes equino varus.

681. An eight-year-old girl presents with a 12-hour history of nausea and central abdominal pain now radiating to the right iliac fossa. She has urinary frequency.

682. A 14-year-old girl has had a pseudomonas urinary tract infection and her blood pressure is 140/95 mmHg persistently. She has a past history of recurrent urinary tract infections and an abdominal ultrasound at the age of two was normal.

Theme Ethical Practice of Medicine in the United Kingdom

Options

A. Report him to trust managers

B. Don't do anything, since the actions of your consultant don't seem to be affecting the progress of patient's condition

C. Call police and inform them at once

D. Give her the pills after explaining risks to her and disregard her mother completely

E. Carry out the termination even without the parents' knowledge

F. Carry out operation to save at least one baby

G. Respect parents decision and let nature take it's course, even if this means certain death for both babies

H. Carry out the sterilization

I. Tell her you cant give her the pills without mothers' consent

J. Give her pills and phone the mother and tell her about the pills

K. Tell the parents and only carry out termination, with their consent

L. Get partners written and informed consent before carrying out sterilisation

M. Inform health minister, as situation is complicated

N. Seek a judicial review

Instructions

For each of the scenarios described below choose the most *appropriate* action from the above group of options.

683. You are the SHO on the Psychiatry ward. Your consultant is having a sexual relationship with a widow he 's been treating for depression. The lady is getting better and is awaiting discharge next week.

684. A 34-year-old woman wants to have a sterilisation .Her last born child has cerebral palsy and her partner strongly objects to the procedure. They are married.

685. A mother has siamese twins. One of the twins has no heart and liver and depends on the other for survival, and as such without an operation to save the one with the major organs they will both perish. Since having the operation means certain death of one the babies, the parents who are staunch Christians oppose the operation. What should be done?

686. A 12-year-old girl wants oral contraceptive pills. She doesn't want her parents to know about this.

687. A 9-year-old girl wants to have a termination of pregnancy. She is 14 weeks pregnant. The procedure to terminate is not without complications. She doesn't want her mother informed about the termination.

Theme Investigation of Confusion

Options

A. Thyroid function tests
B. Blood glucose
C. Mid–stream specimen
D. Computed tomography (CT) scan of head
E. Electrocardiogram (ECG)
F. Full blood count (FBC)
G. Urea and electrolytes
H. Stool culture
I. Blood cultures
J. Ultrasound abdomen
K. Chest X-ray

Instructions

For each presentation below, choose the *single* most discriminating investigation from the above list of options.

Each option may be used once, more than once, or not at all.

688. A 67-year-old man has recently been started on tablets by his GP. He is brought to the Accident and Emergency Department by his wife with sudden onset of aggressive behaviour, confusion and drowsiness. Prior to starting the tablets he was losing weight and complaining of thirst.

689. A 79-year-old man in a nursing home has been constipated for a week. Over the past few days she has become increasingly confused and faecally incontinent.

690. A previously well 70-year-old man has been noticed by her daughter to be increasingly slow and forgetful over several months. She has gained weight and tends to stay indoors with the heating on, even in hot weather.

691. An 80-year-old woman presents with poor mobility and a recent history of fails. She has deteriorated generally over the past two weeks with fluctuating confusion. On examination she has a left hemiplegia.

692. A 70-year-old man with known multiple sclerosis became suddenly more confused yesterday. When seen in the Accident and Emergency Department, his blood pressure was 80/65 mmHg and his pulse was regular at 50/min.

Theme Causes of Maternal Mortality in the United Kingdom

Options

A. First commonest

B. Second commonest

C. Third commonest

D. Fourth commonest

E. Fifth commonest

F. Six commonest

G. Seventh commonest

H. Eighth commonest

Instructions

For each of the conditions mentioned below match them with their corresponding answer, from the list of options above.

693. Acute fatty liver of pregnancy
694. Hypertensive disease of pregnancy
695. Early pregnancy problems eg; ectopics
696. Amniotic fluid embolism
697. Thromboembolism
698. Genital tract sepsis
699. Haemorrhage
700. Uterine rupture

Theme Causes of Perinatal Mortality in the United Kingdom

Options

A. First commonest
B. Second commonest
C. Third commonest
D. Fourth commonest
E. Fifth commonest

Instructions

For each of the conditions below, match them with their corresponding positions, from the list above.

701. Maternal conditions and toxaemia
702. Unclassified hypoxia
703. Congenital abnormalities
704. Placental conditions
705. Cord problems

Theme Prevention/Health Promotion of Fever

Options

A. Tuberculosis
B. Infectious mononucleosis

C. Malaria

D. Gastroenteritis

E. Meningitis

F. Hepatitis A

G. Hepatitis B

H. Hepatitis C

I. Cytomegalo-virus infection

J. Herpes simplex infection

K. Toxoplasmosis

L. Bronchial carcinoma

M. Staphylococcal pneumonia

N. Diptheria

O. Bladder carcinoma

P. Schistosomiasis

Instructions

For each strategy for prevention below, choose the *single* most likely disease to be prevented from the above list of options. Each option may be used once, more than once or not at all.

706. Avoidance of smoking
707. Avoidance of work in dye factories
708. Counselling for sexually active 23-year-old male
709. Prophylaxis with proguanil before travel to Asia
710. Avoidance of swimming in rivers
711. Immunisation of paramedics with body fluids

Theme Risk Factors for the Development of Dementia

Options

A. Postpartum haemorrhage

B. Phenothiazines

C. Decreased CD 4 count

D. Familial inheritance

E. Edwards syndrome

F. Down's syndrome

G. Damage to frontal lobe, and affects women twice as much as men

H. Chronic headache

I. Bartender

J. Klinefelter's syndrome

K. Strokes

L. Childhood meningitis

M. Childhood asphyxia

N. Ingestion of aniline dyes

O. Tainted meat

P. Lewy bodies

Q. Normal pressure hydocephalus

R. Work alcoholics

Instructions

For each of the conditions listed below, choose the *single* most likely risk factor from the list of options above. Each option may be used once, more than once or not at all.

712. AIDS related dementia
713. Alzheimer's disease
714. Multi infarct dementia
715. Parkinson's disease
716. Huntingdon's chorea
717. Diffuse lewy body disease
718. Hypothyroidism
719. Hyperthyroidism
720. Alcoholic dementia
721. Creutzfeldt-Jakob's disease

Theme Diagnosis of Anaemia

Options

A. Sickle cell anaemia

B. Sickle cell trait

C. Sideroblastic anaemia

D. Nutritional anaemia

E. Macrocytic anaemia

F. Microcytosis

G. Iron deficiency anaemia

H. Normochromic normocytic anaemia

I. Aplastic anaemia

Instructions

For each of the patients listed below, choose the *single* most appropriate diagnosis from the list of options above. Each option may be used once, more than once or not at all.

722. A yound Jamaican boy is brought to the Accident and Emergency Department complaining of episodic chest pain associated with pallour. He has a tinge of jaundice.

723. An elderly woman who stays alone is examined by the nurse. She is found to be unkempt with pallour of the mucous membranes.

724. An elderly man lost his wife 10-years ago. He has regular meals but spends most of his time in the 'Old Vic' a, local pub is found to have mild pallour of the mucous membranes.

725. A 24-year-old woman complains of easy fatiguability. Her menses last 7 days and she uses multiple sanitary towels.

726. A 23-year university student travels to Thailand. Days later she complains of abdominal pain and passing bloody watery stools.

Theme Investigation of an Ischaemic Limb

Options

A. Ventilation perfusion (V/Q) scan

B. Electrocardiography (ECG)

C. Ultrasound

D. Femoral duplex scan

E. Femoral arteriography

F. Venography

G. Ankle-brachial index measurement

H. Digital subtraction angiography

I. Coagulation profile

J. None of the above

Instructions

For each of the patients below choose the *single* most definitive investigation from the list of options above. Each option may be used once more than once or not at all.

727. A 36-year-old man complains of pain at rest in his calves.

728. A 34-year-old man complains of pain in the calves on walking. The pain is absent on resting.

729. A 55-year-old man complains of intermittent pain in his toe on walking. He says that in addition it looks 'white'.

730. A 46-year-old woman is brought to the Accident and Emergency Department breathless and complaining of chest pain. He has a two month history of leg pain.

Theme Investigation of Aortic Aneurysm

Options

A. Abdominal Ultrasound
B. Chest X-ray
C. Barium meal
D. Transoesophageal echocardiography
E. Endoscopic studies
F. Barium swallow
G. Computed tomography (CT) scan of head
H. Echocardiography
 I. Spiral computed tomography
 J. Lower limb angiography
K. Coronary angiography
L. Plain abdominal X-ray

Instructions

For each of the patients described below, choose the single most appropriate investigation from the list of options above. Each option may be used once more than once or not at all.

731. A man presents with abdominal pain radiating to the back. He is found to have a pulsatile mass in the abdominal pain. He is haemodynamically stable.

732. A 67-year-old man is being prepared for the repair of an aortic aneurysm. Exercise ECG reveals ischaemia. There is claudication in the legs.

733. This patient is due for repair of aneurysm of aorta, wants to know about the extension of the aneurysm to the renal artery.

734. An obese, 34-year-old man complains of retrosternal pain associated with water brash.

Theme Diagnosis of Shock

Options

A. Anaphylactic shock

B. Neurogenic shock

C. Septic shock

D. Hypovolemic shock

E. Disseminated intravascular coagulation

Instructions

For each of the patients below, choose the *single* most appropriate diagnosis, from the list of options above. Each option may be used once, more than once or not at all.

735. A 64-year-old patient on the surgical ward has been operated on for a hernia, he presents with warm extremities and a blood pressure of 90/60 mmHg.

736. A woman had a ceaserean done in the morning presented with a blood pressure of 80/65 mmHg and pulse rate of 120 beats/min.

737. A 23-year-old man is brought into the Accident and Emergency Department from the local park, with a red swollen arm. He is found to have a blood pressure of 100/60mmHg.

Theme Prognosis of Dementia

Options

A. Alzheimer's disease

B. Cardiovascular accident

C. Lewy body dementia

D. Cataract

E. Parkinsonism

F. Huntingdon's chorea

G. Pick's disease

H. Creutzfeldt-Jakob's disease

Instructions

For each of the patients described below choose the *single* most appropriate diagnosis from the list of options above. Each option may be used once, more than once or not at all.

738. A 57-year-old woman, whose son mentioned that he was becoming progressively forgeting the names of things and chores, was diagnosed 5-7 years ago with dementia, now dies.

739. An elderly woman has a history of episodic weakness of her right arm, all the episodes lasting about 12 hours, is brought by her daughter who says the former, has become progessively forgetful.

740. A 45-year-old man presents with difficulty in initiating movement and general slowness in doing anything. He is put on dopaminergic drugs by his GP but shows no response.

741. A 76-year-old woman is normal at her home, but falls downs at her son's home. She complains of slight blurring of vision. She cannot remember what time of the day she was born.

Theme the Treatment of Burns

Options

A. Admit

B. Irrigation with cold water

C. Application of vaseline

D. Tetanus toxoid

E. Antibiotics

F. Escharotomy

G. Constructive observation combined with debridement

H. Don't admit

Instructions

For each of the scenarios described below, choose the most appropriate action from the list of options above. Each option may be used once.more than once, or not at all.

742. Burns on the anterior chest.

743. Full thickness burns on the genital area.

744. Superficial burns of the right hand, less than 9% of the B.S.A. seen at the moment of injury.

745. A baby with bums, over the chest and back about 7% B.S.A. They are painful.

Theme Differential Diagnosis of Angina

Options

A. Unstable angina

B. Stable angina

C. Syndrome X

D. Myocardial infarction

E. Pericarditis

F. Peptic ulcer disease

G. Arrythmia

H. Spontaneous pneumothorax

I. Acute cholecystitis

J. Chronic cholecystitis

K. Pneumonia

Instructions

For each of the patients below, choose the single most appropriate diagnosis from the list of options above. Each option may be used once, more than once or not at all.

746. An obese 34-year-old man complains of epigastric pain, which seems to exacerbated by eating his favourite meal, fish and chips. He get temporary relief when hungry.

747. An obese 45-year-old man complains of recurring chest pain which radiates to his neck lasting 20 minutes. It coincides with his weekly executive board meetings.

748. An obese 29-year-old woman complains of with a
     cough of two weeks complains of right upper quad-
     rant pain. She is mildly febrile. There was no abdo-
     minal tenderness on examination

Theme Diagnosis of Hypertension

Options

A. Cushing's syndrome

B. Conn's syndrome

C. Pheochromocytoma

D. Essential hypertension

E. Renal artery stenosis

F. Polycystic kidney disease

G. Coarctation of the aorta

Instructions

For each of the patients below, choose the most likely
diagnosis from the list of options above. Each option may
be used once, more than once or not at all.

749. An obese 34-year-old woman presents with excessive
     facial hair, a blood pressure of 150/95 mmHg and
     abdominal striae.

750. A 23-year-old man presents with a chronic headache.
     His blood pressure is 145/90 mmHg. He is found to
     have femoral delay.

751. An elderly man has three readings of blood pressure
     of 160/100 mmHg. He is otherwise well.

752. A 34-year-old man presents with haematuria. His
     blood pressure is found to be 145/100 mmHg. His
     father died from chronic renal failure.

753. A 34-year-old woman presents with intermittent
     flushing, palpitations and headache.

754. A 45-year known hypertensive, is found to have a
     bruit in the abdomen.

Theme Diagnosis of Pelvic Inflammatory Disease

Options

A. Endometriosis

B. Acute chlamydial infection

C. Ectopic pregnancy

D. Gonococcal infection

E. Acute on chronic pelvic inflammatory pelvic disease

F. Chronic pelvic inflammatory disease

G. Abruptio placenta

H. Septic miscarriage

Instructions

For each of the patients below, choose the *single* most appropriate diagnosis from the list of options above. Each option may be used once, more than once or not at all.

755. A 24-year-old university student had a confirmed chlamydial infection 2 years ago. She now presents with acute abdominal pain. Her blood pressure is 90/60 mmHg.

756. A 25-year-old woman who had an Intra-uterine-contraceptive device fitted 2 years ago, presents with heavy per vaginal bleeding. Her pregnancy test is positive.

757. A 24-year-old woman complains of deep dyspareunia. Her periods are regular and her two previous cervical smears were normal.

Theme Investigation of Loss of Consciousness

Options

A. Electroencephalography

B. Ambulatory ECG

C. Exercise ECG

D. Carotid arteriography

E. Computed tomography

F. Echocardiography

G. Do nothing

Instructions

For each of the patients described below, choose the *single* most appropriate diagnosis from the list of options above. Each option may be used once, more than once or not at all.

758. A 12-year-old girl loses consciousness after a period of prolonged standing. She becomes pale but regains consciousness within a few seconds.

759. An elderly woman reports a history of loss of consciousness on five occasions. Each time she regains consciousness after a few minutes.

760. A 34-year-old man has a history of falling with jerky movements of the hands and the feet associated with urinary incontinence.

761. A 12-year-old girl has a history of falling with jerky movements of the body on several occasions. She bites her tongue during the falls.

Theme Management of Septicemia

Options

A. Intravenous catecholamines

B. Intravenous dopamine

C. Intravenous corticosteroids

D. Intravenous dobutamine

E. Oxygen by mask

F. Oral cefuroxamine

G. Stenting

H. Laparotomy and removal of dead tissue

I. Wide excision of soft tissues

J. Percutaneous drainage

Instructions

For each of the patients described below, choose the most appropriate management from the list of options above. Each option may be used once, more than once or not at all.

762. A 28-year-old woman after cholecystectomy following a perforated gall bladder has a raised right diaphragm with a temperature of 38°C and a pulse of 120 beats per minute.

763. A febrile 39-year-old woman with hypertension, has a history of recurrent urinary tract infections. Abdominal ultra sound showed a dilated calyx.

764. A 32-year-old woman has chickenpox. She scratches herself excessively and develops a blue discoloration on the abdomen. She has a history of not passing urine in the last 24 hours. She continues to scratch herself and the discolouration increases in size.

Theme Diagnosis of Neurological Abnormalities

Options

A. Vertebro-basilar infarction

B. Cerebral infarct

C. Subarachnoid haemorrhage

D. Cerebral haemorrhage

E. Hypoglycaemia

F. Cerebello pontine haemorrhage

G. Hypercalcemia

H. Multiple sclerosis

I. Polymyalgia rheumatica

Instructions

For each of the patients described below choose the *single* most likely cause of their symptoms and signs from the list of options above. Each option may be used once, more than once or not at all.

765. An elderly man wakes up in the morning with numbness of his right hand, blurring of vision in his right eye. He then suffers a drop attack.

766. A 33-year-old man reports a history of walking while swinging to one side.

767. A 32-year-old known hypertensive presents to you with a right hemiparesis.

768. A 34-year-old woman has a 6 months history of on and off hemiparesis which resolves with no neurological deficits.

769. A 55-year-old woman treated for breast cancer with chemotherapy and radiotherapy presented with a history of confusion, tiredness, weakness and poyuria. On examination no neurological deficits were found.

Theme Diagnosis of
Lower Gastrointestinal Bleeding

Options

A. Ulcerative colitis

B. Amoebic dysentery

C. Crohn's disease

D. Carcinoma of the rectum

E. Carcinoma of the sigmoid

F. Diverticular disease

G. Diverticulosis

H. Ulcerative pancolitis

 I. Trauma

J. Tuberculous enteritis

K. HIV enteropathy

Instructions

For each of the patients described below,choose the *single* most likely cause of lower GIT bleeding from the list of options above. Each option may be used once, more than once or not at all.

770. A young man presents with abdominal pain,bleeding per rectum. Barium enema reveals an ulcerated stricture of the sigmoid colon.

771. A young man presents with per rectal bleeding. Investigation shows granular inflammation in the distal 12 cm of the sigmoid colon. The proximal area is normal.

772. A young woman with per rectal bleeding is found to have ulcers in the anal area and vulva. Colonoscopy revealed ulcers in the transverse colon.

773. A 45-year-old man presents with abdominal pain, frequent stools (about 5 episodes a day). He denied they were blood stained and barium studies show a filling defect in the ascending colon. His Hb was 8g/dl, MCV 67 fl.

Theme Diagnosis of Visual Loss

Options

A. Acute glaucoma

B. Central retinal vein occlusion

C. Central retinal artery occlusion

D. Cranial arteritis

E. Uveitis

F. Occipital lobal infarct

G. Direct trauma

H. Retrobulbar neuritis

I. Retinal detachment

Instructions

For each of the patients described below, choose the *single* most likely cause of visual loss from the list of options above. Each option may be used once, more than once or not at all.

774. A 35-year-old man presents with pain in the right eye, vomiting and loss of vision.

775. A 55-year-old known diabetic and hypertensive wakes up in the morning with diminished vision

776. A 25-year-old man presents to the Accident and Emergency Department with pain in the right eye associated with backache.

777. An elderly woman presents with a history of visual loss and scalp soreness.

778. An elderly man who is an in-patient (for hypertension) wakes in the morning notes that he can't see his breakfast. He has no other complaints. He has a carotid bruit.

Theme Investigation of Chronic Joint Pain

Options

A. Joint aspiration and culture
B. X-ray of the joint
C. Aspirate for monourate crystals
D. ESR
E. Rheumatoid factor
F. Weakly positive birefringent crystals
G. Urinalysis
H. Computed tomography
I. Fine needle aspiration cytology

Instructions

For each of the patients described below, choose the *single* most appropriate investigation from the list of options above. Each option may be used once, more than once or not at all.

779. A 53-year-old woman presents with on and off left knee pain. On examination it's found to be swollen. She also complains stiffness in the hands and feet especially in the morning.

780. A 60-year-old woman presents with pain in her right hip, most marked at rest and at the end of the day associated with mild stiffness and joint instability.

781. A 73-year-old fit farmer presents with a painful, swollen and hot right wrist. He has a fever and general malaise.

782. An elderly woman started on diuretics three weeks ago now presents with a red hot swollen metatarsal phalangeal joint.

Theme Management of Varicose Veins

Options

A. Graduated compression stockings
B. Crepe bandage
C. X-ray

D. Skin graft

E. Doppler ultrasound

F. Elevation of the leg

G. Sclerosant

H. Lose weight

Instructions

For each of the patients described below, choose the *single* most appropriate answer from the list of options above. Each option may be used once, more than once or not at all.

783. A middle aged man with bilateral leg varicose veins is to fly to New York for a business meeting. He comes to you for advice. His father died of embolism. He is scared of surgical operations.

784. An obese woman has bilateral leg varicose veins. Her BMI is 30 and she is found to have lipodermosclerosis around her shins.

785. A 54-year-old man presented with varicose veins which developed following a compound fracture of the left lower limb a couple of weeks ago and have persisted.

786. A 45-year-old woman with a BMI of 33 presents with bilateral varicose veins. No treatment has been attempted.

Theme Complications of Blood Dyscrasia

Options

A. Generalised lymphadenopathy

B. Meningitis

C. Massive splenomegaly

D. Purpura

E. Bone Pain

F. Gum hyperplasia

G. Thrombophilia

Instructions

For each of the patients described below, choose the *single* most likely complication from the list above. Each option may be used once, more than once or not at all.

787. A 34-year-old woman with increased granulocyte series and a raised platelet count.
788. A young boy with cervical lymphadenopathy and a raised white blood cell count.
789. A 3-year-old boy presents with neck stifiness, photo-phobia and headache. Blood film shows a marked lymphocytosis.
790. A 38-year-old woman presents with cervical lymph-adenopathy. Mature lymphoblasts are seen on the blood film. Examination reveals a mild splenomegaly. He is on phenytoin for epilepsy.

Theme Diagnosis of Earache

Options

A. Otitis media
B. Otitis externa
C. Herpes zoster
D. Temporal mandibular joint disease
E. Acoustic neuroma
F. Perforation of the ear drum
G. Mumps
H. Glue ear
I. Mastoiditis
J. Dental caries

Instructions

For each of the patients described below, choose the *single* most likely diagnosis from the list of options above. Each option may be used once, more than once or not at all.

791. A 23-year-old avid swimmer develops an ear dis-charge and inflammation on the pinna.
792. A 12-year-old boy presents with earache. On exami-nation, there is a swelling extending from the ear to the angle of the jaw.
793. An elderly man on chemotherapy for colonic cancer develops pain in the right ear. On examination, the right ear is found to have vesicles. He later develops weakness on the right side of the body.

794. A 56-year-old woman complains of earache, worsened by stress. On opening her mouth 'noises' are heard. Her husband says she tends to grind her teeth at night.

795. A 15-year-old boy with a history of right earache now presents with a right ear discharge. The pain has abated.

Theme Investigation of Diabetes

Options

A. Random blood sugar
B. Glucose tolerance test
C. Urea and electrolytes
D. 24 hour urinary free cortisol
E. Dexamethasone suppression test
F. Serum amylase
G. Synacthen test
H. Ultrasound of the abdomen
I. X-ray of the abdomen
J. Abdominal computed tomgraphy

Instructions

For each of the patients described below, choose the most appropriate test from the list of options above. Each option may be used once, more than once or not at all.

796. A known diabetic presents with dehydration, deep sighing respiration, sweet smelling breath and altered consciousness. Blood sugar is 27 mmol/l.

797. A 29-year-old woman presents with polyuria and polydipsia. She is found to have a 'moon' face, truncal obesity and is easily bruised. Blood sugar is 15 mmol/L.

798. A 40-year-old woman presents with dehydration. She has a history of polyuria, polydipsia. Blood glucose is 7 mmol/L. She has chronic pancreatitis.

799. An obese woman presents with polyuria and polydipsia, but is otherwise well.

Theme Diagnosis of Breathlessness

Options

A. Fibrosing alveolitis
B. Occupational lung disease
C. Extrinsic allergic alveolitis
D. Allergic bronchopulmonary aspergillosis
E. Asthma
F. Pneumonia
G. Bronchiectasis
H. Pulmonary tuberculosis

Instructions

For each of the patients described below, choose the *single* most likely diagnosis from the list of options above. Each option may be used once, more than once or not at all.

800. A farmer who keeps pigeons develops breathlessness, which progressively worsens and later resolves on its own, spirometry shows a restrictive pattern.
801. A coal miner develops progressives breathlessness.
802. A young boy is diagnosed with asthma and is started on inhaled bronchodilators. He is getting worse despite treatment and the parents are getting concerned. Serum IgE is raised.
803. A 7-year-old boy had measles 2-years ago, now presents with a productive cough associated with occasional haemoptysis.

Theme Diagnosis of Chest Pain

Options

A. Chest X-ray
B. Exercise ECG
C. Echocardiography
D. Gastroscopy
E. Oesophagoscopy

F. Computed tomography

G. ECG

H. Pulmonary angiography

I. Cardiac catheterization

J. Indirect laryngoscopy

Instructions

For each of the patients described below, choose the *single* most likely diagnosis from the list of options above. Each option may be used once, more than once or not at all.

804. A 30-year-old obese man complains of retrosternal chest pain, worse at night and after meals.

805. A 34-year-old man presents with a history of chest pain radiating to the jaw, brought on by exercise and relieved by rest.

806. A 67-year-old woman presents with a 2-hour history of chest pain radiating to the left shoulder. He is sweating and feels sick.

807. A tall young man presents with a history of sudden chest pain radiating to the back and interscapular area.

Theme Management of a Rash

Options

A. Isolation/quarantine

B. Reassure

C. Acyclovir

D. Hydrocortisone cream

E. PUVA

F. A half day course of rifampicin

G. Immunize against measles

H. Check anticardiolipin antibodies

Instructions

For each of the patients described below, choose the *single* most appropriate option, from the list of options above. Each option may be used once, more than once or not at all.

808. A distressed mother rings you. She's found out that one of the children at her daughters school has meningitis.

809. A pregnant woman gets a transient rash which disappears. The young woman is otherwise well.

810. A boy with a vesicular rash and fever goes to his GP. His sister has just been discharged following a renal transplant.

Theme Trauma and Oliguria

Options

A. Percutaneuos nephrostomy

B. Suprapubic cystostomy

C. Urethral catheterization

D. Blood transfusion

E. Fluid challenge

F. 500 ml of IV mannitol

G. Walk around

Instructions

For each of the patients below, choose the most appropriate option from the list of options above. Each option may be used once more than once or not at all.

811. Following an elective herniorrhaphy, a 67-year-old man is unable to pass urine, when a nurse hands him a small bottle for microscopic studies. He is otherwise well.

812. A 34-year-old woman presents with right sided loin pain and oliguria. An intravenous urogram shows right sided dilated calyces and hydroureter.

813. A man involved in a mining accident presents with oliguria and passing dark brown urine.

814. A 45-year-old man sustained a pelvic fracture and now presents with oliguria, a pulse rate of 120 beats/min and a blood pressure of 70/50 mmHg.

815. A 23-year-old man who sustained a pelvic fracture is unable to pass urine. On examination he has abdominal tenderness and fullness and blood on the urethral meatus.

Theme Prenatal Diagnosis

Options

A. Cordocentesis

B. Rhesus status

C. Kleihauer test

D. Chorionic villus sampling

E. Abdominal ultrasound

F. Biophysical profile

G. Amniocentesis

Instructions

For each of the patients described below, choose the *single* most appropriate option, from the list of options above. Each option may be used once, more than once or not at all.

816. A 23-year-old primigravida at 13 weeks, is told after screening that she has a 75% chance of getting a baby with Down's syndrome. She wants to know whether her child actually has the syndrome.

817. A 25-year-old pregnant sickler wants to know whether her baby will have the haemoglobinopathy.

818. A 30-week pregnant woman had an episode of antepartum haemorrhage during the current pregnancy. A detailed ultrasound shows a grossly retarded foetus, but with no physical abnormality.

819. A 33-year-old rhesus negative woman had isoimmunisation in her last pregnancy. A biophysical profile shows an oedematous foetus.

Theme Management of Pain in Labour

Options

A. Spinal anaesthesia

B. Epidural anaesthesia

C. Pudendal nerve block

D. General anaesthesia

E. Pethidine injection

F. Nitrous oxide

G. Local anaesthesia

Instructions

For each of the patients described below, choose the most appropriate option, from the list of options above. Each option may be used once, more than once or not at all.

820. A 20-year-old primigravida at 40-weeks, is 6 cm is dilated and she requests pain relief. She dislikes injections.

821. A 39-year gravida 3 para 2 + 0, presents at 39-weeks. Her cervix is 8 cm dilated but she complains of severe pain. Her baby is in occipitoposterior position.

822. A 28-year-old woman wants to be able to move around during labour, pain free.

823. A Gravida 4 para 2 + l, has been in labour for 4 hours. She is 3 cm dilated and has already received 2 injections of pethidine. She stills complains of pain.

824. A 31-year-old woman has a retained placenta, following a spontaneous vaginal delivery.

Theme Pelvic Inflammatory Disease

Options

A. Acute PID

B. Acute on chronic PID

C. Gonorrhoea

D. Bacterial vaginosis

E. Lymphogranuloma venerum

F. Ectopic pregnancy

G. Threatened miscarriage

H. Toxic shock syndrome

I. Syphilis

J. Chronic PID

Instructions

For each of the patients described below choose the *single* most appropriate answer from the list of options above. Each option may be used once, more than once or not at all.

825. A 24-year-old woman is in her periods. She now presents with fever (38ºC) and a foul smelling vaginal discharge and a blood pressure of 100/65 mmHg.

826. A 24-year woman presents with a foul smelling vaginal discharge.

827. A 34-year-old woman with a history of pelvic inflammatory disease, now presents with deep dyspareunia and pain in the lower abdomen.

828. A 32-year-old woman with an Intra-uterine device complains of right iliac fossa pain, amenorrhoea for the 6-weeks.

829. A 33-year woman with a history of pelvic inflammatory disease, now presents with lower abdominal pain and fever (38ºC).

Theme the Disease Process of Asthma

Options

A. 5% reversibility in FEV_1

B. 10% reversibility in FEV_1

C. 15% reversibility in FEV_1

D. Alpha receptors

E. Beta 2 receptors

F. Eosinophils

G. Forced vital capacity

H. Histamine

I. IgA

J. IgE

K. IgG

L. IgM

M. Leukotrienes

N. Mast cells

O. Neutrophils

P. Peak expiratory flow rate (PEFR)

Q. Positive pollen test

R. Raised eosinophil count

S. T cells

T. Vital capacity

Instructions

For each of the statements below, choose the *single* most likely connecting statement from the above list of options. Each option may be used once, more than once or not at all.

830. A criterion for the diagnosis of asthma.
831. The substance is released by mast cell activation and causes bronchospasm.
832. Found commonly in the sputum of patients with asthma.
833. Blocking of these can cause worsening of asthma.

Theme Diagnosis of Hip pain

Options

A. Fracture neck of femur
B. Perthes disease
C. Slipped femoral epiphysis
D. Osteoarthritis
E. Septic arthritis
F. Congenital dislocation of the hip
G. Transient synovitis
H. Osteogenesis imperfecta

Instructions

For each of the patients described below, choose the *single* most likely diagnosis from the list of options above. Each option may be used once, more than once or not at all.

834. A 7-year boy presents with a history of acute onset of pain in the knee. On examination, the left lower limb is flexed, abducted, internally rotated.
835. A 67-year-old woman complains of right hip pain. On examination the right hip is adducted, externally rotated and flexed.
836. A 10-year-old girl is febrile. On examination it's difficult to abduct the thighs.
837. A child presents with right hip pain. On examination the hip is flexed, abducted and externally rotated.

Theme Diagnosis of Central Chest Pain

Options

A. Myocardial infarction
B. Oesophageal candidiasis
C. CMV oesophagitis
D. Reflux oesophagitis
E. Tietze's syndrome
F. Acute cholecystitis
G. Peptic ulcer disease
H. Constrictive pericarditis
I. Pulmonary embolism
J. Angina pectoris
K. Dissecting aortic aneurysm

Instructions

For each of the patients described below, choose the *single* most likely diagnosis from the list of options above. Each option may be used once, more than once or not at all.

838. A thin 60-year-old man presents with a 2-hour history of a crushing central chest pain.

839. A 40-year-old man with a history of high blood pressure presents with central chest pain radiating to the interscapular area.

840. A young homosexual man complains of central chest pain. On examination of his mouth, he has white granular lesions on the buccal mucosa which is red.

841. A 20-year-old man with a history of drug abuse presents with sudden onset central chest pain associated with passage of maelena stool.

842. A 60-year-old woman with a history of calf pain following an anterior resection of the rectum presents with sudden onset central chest pain.

Theme Treatment of Arrythmias

Options

A. Fleicanide

B. Amiodarone

C. Chloroquine

D. Digoxin

E. Temporary pacing

F. Permanent pacing

G. DC cardioversion

H. Lignocaine

I. Reassurance

J. Nifedipine

K. Glyceryl trinitrate

L. Warfarin

M. 5 ml of a 1:1000 solution of Adrenaline

N. Atropine

Instructions

For each of the patients below choose the *single* most appropriate intervention from the list of options above. Each option may be used once, more than once or not at all.

843. A 20-year-old officer worker gets palpitations whenever he walks a flight of several stairs to work.

844. A 55-year-old man complains of chest pain. His Blood pressure is 145/92 mmHg. His pulse is irregularly irregular.

845. A 55-year-old man presents with dyspnoea and chest pain. He is found to have a broad complex tachycardia on ECG.

846. A 68-year-old man found to have a pulse rate of 60 beats/min and complains of chest pain and breathlessness. Drug treatment is no help.

847. A 69-year-old man is complains of chest pain. He has had previous episodes of severe bradycardia, cardiac arrest, and supraventricular tachycardias alternating with asystole.

848. Useful for the conversion a supraventricular tachy-cardia to sinus rythmn, if done in synchrony with the QRS complex.

849. A 45-year-old man presents with dyspnoea and chest pain. The ECG shows a short PR interval and wide QRS which begins with a 'slurred' upstroke (delta wave)

Theme Treatment of Ear Infections

Options

A. Chloramphenicol ear drops

B. Amoxycillin

C. Amoxycillin and clavulanic acid

D. Penicillin

E. Cefllroxime

F. Ear wash out

G. Syringing

H. Removal with forceps

Instructions

For each of the patients described below, choose the *single* most appropriate answer from the list of options above. Each option may be used once, more than once or not at all.

850. A 13-year-old boy complains or a headache. Otoscopy reveals a right perforated ear drum with a purulent discharge.

851. A 7-year-old girl complains of right earache. Examination reveals a bulging hyperaemic right ear-drum. The left eardrum looks grey.

852. A 14-year-old girl complains of diminished hearing in the right ear. Otoscopy shows waxy material in the canal.

853. A 4-year-old boy with a fever is found to have a bead in his left ear.

854. A 24-year-old woman has a purulent lesion in her right canal. She has a fever and doesn't complain of hearing loss.

Theme Treatment of UTI in Children

Options

A. Trimethoprim l-2 mg/kg/single dose

B. Trimethoprim 3 mg /kg/bd

C. Amoxycillin

D. Amoxycillin 500 mg/8hr

E. Gentamicin 10 mg/kg/day

F. Nitrafurantoin 12 mg/kg/day

G. Ciprofloxacillin 500 mg stat

H. Metronidazole 500 mg/kg/day

I. Co-amoxiclav 20-45 mg/kg/day

J. Nalidixic acid 50 mg/kg/day

Instructions

For each of the patients listed below, choose the *single* most appropriate treament from the list of options above. Each option may be used once, more than once or not all.

855. A 2-year-old boy is with frequency and dysuria shown to have vesico-ureteric reflux. He is treated for the acute infection and you want him to stay healthy until surgical intervention.

856. A 6-year-old girl presents with a fever, frequency dysuria and abdominal pain.

857. A 5-year-old boy presents with dysuria, fever, frequency and vomiting. Abdominal ultrasound shows no abnormalities.

858. Almost 50% of all *e. coli* infections are now unresponsive to this.

Theme Poisoning

Options

A. Aspirin

B. Atropine

C. Paracetamol

D. Iron

E. Morphine

F. Warfarin

G. Carbon monoxide

H. Oxygen

I. Quinine

J. Corticosteroids

Instructions

For each of the scenarios below, choose the most appropriate intervention/aetiology. Each option may be used once, more than once or not at all.

859. Desferrioxamine is used in poisoning.

860. Patient presents within urinary retention, dry mouth and sedation. What is the possible aetiological agent?

861. A 24-year-old took an overdose of pills and now complains of right upper quadrant pain. He is found to be hypoglycemic.

Theme Diagnosis of Vaginal Discharge in Children

Options

A. Foreign body

B. Candidiasis

C. Physiological

D. Bacterial vaginosis

E. Trichomonas vaginalis

F. Sexual abuse

G. Urinary tract infection

H. Gonorrhoea

I. Threadworm infection

K. Juvenile cervical carcinoma

Instructions

For each of the patients below, choose the *single* most likely diagnosis from the list of options above. Each option may be used once, more than once or not at all.

862. A sexually active 13-year-old girl presents with a mild non-fouling smelling vaginal discharge.

---

863. A 6-year-old girl is brought with a fouling smelling vaginal discharge. There is no history of sexual abuse.
864. A 5-year-old girl who is in foster care is noted to have a foul smelling vaginal discharge. She is under-weight.
865. A 12-year-old girl who under went a renal transplant 4 months ago presents with a white curdly vaginal discharge.

Theme Management of Dementia

Options

A. Benzhexol
B. levodopa
C. Dopamine
D. Mannitol
E. Dexamethasone
F. 50 ml of 50% glucose
G. Immunoglobulin
H. Donezepil
I. Try shunting
J. Multi-vitamins

Instructions

For each of the patients described below, choose the *single* most appropriate treatment from the list of options above. Each option may be used once, more than once or not at all.

866. A 59-year-old man with no previous history brought by his wife who says he has become progressively more forgetful, tends to lose his temper and emotionally labile. There is no history of infectious disease or trauma.
867. A 43-year-old woman presents with memory loss, poor concentration and inability to recognise household objects. She has drooling and a mask-like face.
868. A 67-year-old man presents with increased forgetfulness, urinary incontinence. Investigations reveal normal CSF pressure and constituents with enlarged cerebral ventricles and no cortical atrophy.
869. A 67-year-old man has been a bartender for 30 years. He has become increasingly forgetful and emotionally labile.

Theme: Pharmacology and Toxicology

Options

A. Tricyliantidepressants

B. Opiate

C . Naloxone

D. Warfarin

E. Specific antidote

F. Heparin

G. Cyanide

H. Ethanol

 I. Vitamin A

 J. Paracetamol

K. 100% O_2

Instructions

Choose the most appropriate.

870. A homeless patient presents to A and E with drowsiness. On examination, abrasions and puncture marks were found on his arm. What would you give?

871. This drug competes with vitamin K.

872. A man was found in his car with a hose directed from the exhaust. What would you give?

873. A patient who has overdosed on an unknown medication presents with palpitations. What is the most likely cause?

874. This interferes with metabolism at the mitochondrial level.

875. This drug in overdose is treated with N-acetylcysteine.

Theme: Management of Meningitis

Options

A. Lumbar Puncture

B. Blood transfusion

C. Steroids

D. Reassure and discharge

E. IV benzylpenicillin

F. Fresh frozen plasma

G. Prophylaxis of contacts

Instructions

Choose the most appropriate.

876. A child of 8-year-old was brought to A and E with headache and neck stiffness. Fundoscopy revealed papilloedema. Blood pressure is high.

877. A child with neck stiffness, drowsiness and purpuric rash over his body.

878. A child with fever, headache and neck stiffness was given IV penicillin. He has recovered in the ward and all his vital signs are stable. What would you like to do now?

Theme: Diagnosis of Dementia

Options

A. Alzheimer's disease

B. Prion disease

C. Huntington's disease

D. Multiple sclerosis

E. Parkinson's disease

F. Multi-infarct dementia

G. Alcohol-related dementia

H. Old age

Instructions

Choose the most appropriate.

879. This dementia may appear in the middle aged and develop in a step-wise fashion.

880. This dementia usually appears late in life and it is progressive.

881. This dementia may lead to death within 10 years.

882. The onset of this dementia is insidious with gradual deterioration.

883. A young man with behavioural changes. There is a history of similar condition in his family.

Theme: Diagnosis of Arrhythmias

Options

A. Ventricular fibrillation

B. Third degree block

C. Wenckebach-type block

D. Paroxysmal atrial fibrillation

E. Atrial flutter

F. Supraventricular tachycardia

G. Ectopics

Instructions

Choose the most appropriate.

884. A woman complains of palpitations during the day. She says it usually starts when she falls to sleep. She describes the feeling that her heart misses a beat from time to time.

885. A man presents with palpitations. It responded well to Carotid Sinus Massage.

Theme: Management of Agitation

Options

A. Counselling

B. Psychotherapy

C. Reassure

D. IM antipsychotics

E Cognitive therapy

F. Admit to hospital

G. IV diazepam

H. Tricyclic antidepressants

Instructions

Choose the most appropriate.

886. A man is brought to A and E with agitation. He had history of attempted suicide twice before. This time he is threatening to kill himself after going home.

887. An agitated schizophrenic is attempting suicide.
888. A man on the second post-operative day is attacking the nurses and wants to jump from the window.

Theme: Causes of Pneumonia

Options

A Klebsiella
B *Mycoplasma pneumoniae*
C *Pneumocystis carinii*
D Mycobacterium TB
E Bronchiectasis
F Streptococcus pneumoniae
G Haemophilus influenzae

Instructions

Choose the most appropriate.

889. An 18-year-old student recently joined university. He suffers from fever, cough and malaise. Amoxicillin showed no response.
890. 35-year-old woman presenting with four-month history of productive cough, night sweats and on occasions haemoptysis. She also has considerable weight loss.
891. 28-year-old man presenting with cough, producing frothy, foul smelling sputum. Chest X-ray shows multiple small cavities.
892. A prostitute complains of increased cough and fever. Chest X-ray shows peri-hilar fine mottling.
893. 60-year-old man was treated for fever, cough, malaise and the symptoms resolved. Three weeks later CXR was taken in the OPD and showed lobar consolidation.

Theme: Treatment of Acute Pain

Options

A. IV morphine and O_2
B. IV morphine
C IM diclofenac

D Distraction

E Sugar sweetened feed

F Local anaesthetic

G Indomethacin orally for one week

Instructions

Choose the most appropriate.

894. 50-year-old man presenting to the A and E with severe retrosternal chest pain radiating to the left arm. He has suffered pain for 30 minutes.

895. A middle-aged man presents to the A and E with severe pain in the loin.

896. 6-year-old girl needs a urinary catheter to be inserted.

897. Patient with renal failure complains of pain in the first metatarso-phalangeal joint.

Theme: Investigation of Hoarse Voice

Options

A. Larynoscopy

B. No need to investigate immediately

C. Throat swab

D. Blood culture

E. Paul-Bunnell test

Instructions

Choose the most appropriate.

898. A singer complains of a hoarse voice for the last three weeks.

899. A young man develops a hoarse voice after a football match.

900. 5-year-old child develops a fever, cough, hoarse voice and the cervical lymph nodes are enlarged.

Theme: Causes of Visual Disturbance

Options

A. Pituitary tumour

B. Acute glaucoma

C. Amaurosis fugax

D. Retinal detachment

E. Occipital lobe infarction

Instructions

Choose the most appropriate.

901. A 50-year-old man complains of loss of vision in one eye, which resolved after 15 minutes.

902. A man has gradual onset of headache, tunnel vision and bitemporal hemianopia.

Theme: Investigation of Confusion

Options

A. Blood glucose

B. Chest X-ray

C. Stool culture

D. Ultrasound abdomen

E. CT scan of head

F. Blood culture

G. ECG

H. Mid stream specimen of urine

I. Full blood count

J. Thyroid function tests

Instructions

Choose the most appropriate.

903. 84-year-old in a nursing home has been constipated for a week. She has become increasingly confused and incontinent

904. A 78-year-old woman has been noticed by her daughter to be increasingly slow and forgetful over several months. She has gained weight and tends to stay indoors with the heating on in the warm weather.

905. 64-year-old man recently started on tablets by his G.P. He is brought to A and E by his wife with sudden onset of aggressive behaviour, confusion and drowsiness. Prior to starting the tablets he was losing weight and complaining of thirst.

906. A frail 85-year-old woman present with poor mobility and a recent history of falls. She has generally deteriorated over the past two weeks with fluctuating confusion. On examination she has mild right hemiparesis.

907. 75-year-old man with known Alzheimer's disease became suddenly more confused yesterday. When seen in A and E his BP was 90/60. His pulse was 40 beats/min and regular.

Theme: Diagnosis of Dysphagia

Options

A. Cancer of oesophagus
B. Achalasia of the cardia
C. Oesophageal stricture
D. Oesophageal candidiasis
E. Pharyngeal pouch
F. Motor neurone disease

Instructions

Choose the most appropriate.

908. A 28-year-old homosexual man complains of difficulty and pain during swallowing.

909. 65-year-old man develops dysphagia, malaise over a period of eight weeks. He shows more than a 10Kg weight toss during this time.

910. 58-year-old man complains of difficulty to swallow especially after his first meal. He also gives a history of repeated chest infections and food regurgitating in the night.

911. A 48-year-old woman presents with a two-year history of progressive dysphagia of solids and liquids. She also suffers from recurrent chest infections.

Theme: Haematemesis and Melaena

Options

A. Duodenal ulcer
B. Gastric ulcer
C. Oesophageal ulcer

D. Oesophageal varices

E. Mallory-weiss syndrome

F. Hereditary haemorrhagic telangiectasia

Instructions

Choose the most appropriate.

912. A 19-year-old suffers profuse vomiting after excessive drinking of alcohol in one evening. The vomit is mixed with small amounts of fresh blood.

Theme: Diagnosis of Skin Disorders

Options

A. Urticaria

B Psoriasis

C Eczema

D Pemphigoid

E Lichen planus

F. Henoch-Schonlein purpura

G. Pemphigus

H. Contact dermatitis

I. Scabies

Instructions

Choose the most appropriate.

913. A 20-year-old girl presents with purple spots on her buttocks and outer forearms. She also has pain in her joints and abdomen. Urine test shows proteinuria.

914. A patient presents with itchy lesions on the wrists, ···hich is associated with fine lacy patches on her ... ·cal mucosa.

Theme: Investigation of Lung Disease: Most Definitive Test

Options

. Chest X-ray

Bronchoscopy and biopsy

C. Sputum microscopy and culture

D. Pleural biopsy

Instructions

Choose the most appropriate.

915. A 20-year-old woman has a three-day history of fever, cough and breathlessness.

916. A 35-year-old Asian woman has a one-month history of cough, fever and night sweats.

Theme: Causes of Neck and Back Pain

Options

A. Torticollis

B. Whiplash injury

C. Multiple myeloma

D. Osteoarthritis

E. Prolapsed intervertebral disc

F. Ankylosing spondylitis

Instructions

Choose the most appropriate.

917. A 35-year-old man presents with sudden pain in his lower back while lifting a heavy load. The pain radiates down his right leg.

918. A young man presents with a one-day history of pain and stiffness in his neck. The previous day he had been a passenger in a car that had been involved in a minor accident.

Theme: Causes of Hand Abnormalities

Options

A. Radial nerve palsy

B. Dupuytren's contracture

C. Syringomyelia

D. Ulnar nerve palsy

E. Median nerve palsy

F. Peripheral neuropathy

G. Brachial plexus injury

Instructions

Choose the most appropriate.

919. A patient presents with a history of progressive inability to extend his ring and little fingers, which are held in fixed flexion.

920. A man complains of paraesthesiae, impaired sensation to light, touch and vibration affecting all the digits of both hands.

Theme: The Diagnosis of Neurological Complaints

Options

A. Diabetes mellitus

B. Vitamin B deficiency

C. Depression

D. Myasthenia gravis

E. Syringomyelia

F. Botulism

G. Lead poisoning

H. Discoid lupus erythematosus

I. Systemic lupus erythematosus

J. Cerebrovasuclar accident

K. Aortic aneurysm

L. Leprosy

M. Dermatomyositis

N. Polymyositis

Instructions

Choose an option from the list of diagnoses given above that is most likely for the individual presentations given below. You may use each option once, more than once, or not at all.

921. An elderly man who tins his own foods suffers from blurred vision, photophobia, and spasticity. He

complains of difficulty speaking and is brought in by his son. His breathing is laboured.

922. A young adult complains about loss of sensation and temperature, especially in the neck and shoulders. Recently, he has injured his arm and hands quite badly without feeling anything.

923. A middle aged woman presents with recurrent nausea, weight loss, and fever. She has pain, stiffness, and weakness in her hips, and shoulders. She does not have a rash, but the skin around the neck and shoulders appears thickened.

924. A 48-year-old man complains of ill health, joint pain, and muscle weakness. He has a fever, loss of appetite, nausea, and weight loss. The patient points to a circular area of white and thickened skin behind his ear. He says the hair has never grown back.

925. A 28-year-old student complains of exhaustion. Studying into the night causes his eyes to twitch and his head to become heavy. He is very easily fatigued and can not carry on with his ordinary chores as usual.

Theme: The Diagnosis of Facial Pain

Options

A. Migraine

B. Abscess

C. Coryza

D. Serous otitis media

E. Glaucoma

F. Iritis

G. Trigeminal neuralgia

H. Sinusitis

I. Systemic lupus erythematosus

J. Head lice

K. Herpes zoster

L. Space occupying lesion

M. Meningitis

N. Temporal arteritis

Instructions

Examine the following five cases of facial pain and decide which of the above mentioned diagnoses is most likely given the somewhat limited information you have before you. You may use each diagnosis once, more than once, or not at all.

926. A 53-year-old nurse complains of facial pain. A week earlier she had a red rash and blisters around her right eye. This area of her face has now become acutely painful.

927. A 31-year-old man complains of facial pain between the eyes and on one side of the face. His nose and the affected eye are congested. He says the pain is severe.

928. A 20-year-old man says his face hurts, especially around the eyes and cheeks. When he bends forwards it worsens and makes him cry.

929. A 57-year-old teacher says she has facial pain, especially in the temples at night. On the right side of her face it throbs. For the past three weeks she has felt unwell and had to miss classes. Also, combing her hair has become painful.

930. A 43-year-old mechanic complains of left sided facial pain. The pain is stabbing and runs up and down his face, especially at meal times. He has been to the dentist, but the dentist has found his teeth to be in good order.

Theme: The Diagnosis of Difficulties with Micturition

Options

A. Preganacy
B. Infection
C. Gylcosuria
D. Congenital abnormalities
E. Bladder tumour
F. Childbirth
G. Crohn's disease
    Urge incontinence
    Stress incontinence

J. True incontinence

K. Vesico-vaginal fistula

L. Urethral syndrome

M. Gonorrhoea

N. Tuberculosis

Instructions

For each of the patient cases given below choose an appropriate and accurate diagnosis from the list of options given above. You may use each options once, more than once, or not at all.

931. An overweight woman complains of having to go to the toilet more than usual. She says she does drink a lot of tea but that she is always thirsty and tired. She needs the energy.

932. A young mother with chronic bronchitis says that every time she coughs, she pees, and she would like you to do something about it. She is on a course of antibiotics at the moment.

933. A middle aged woman complains of having to urinate frequently. She says that unless she rushes to the toilet she wets herself and she finds wetting herself most embarrassing.

934. A 36-year-old sales executive says she wets herself without warning. Before the birth of her third child she had no complaints but now she says she has no control whatsoever.

935. A 27-year-old travel guide wants something done about the pain she feels on micturition, especially when it is cold. Repeated urine cultures have all been negative. Sometimes, she says, going to the toilet is very painful for her.

Theme: The Management of Abdominal Pain

Options

A. Food poisoning

B. Alcohol poisoning

C. Epilepsy

D. Trauma

E. Space occupying lesion

F. Cerebral malaria

G. Enteric fever

H. Lead poisoning

I. Phaeochromacytoma

J. Renal failure

K. Meningitis

L. Dessminated intravascular coagulation

M. Aspirin poisoning

N. Diamorphine overdose

Instructions

From the list of options given above choose the diagnosis that most fully and accurately reflects the details of the individual presentations given below. You may use each option once, more than once, or not at all.

936. A young woman is found unconscious. On examination of her eyes you find pin point pupils. Her body temperature is low.

937. An adolescent boy develops a high fever and collapses unconscious. On physical examination you find a purpuric rash.

938. A businessman recently returned from Malaysia is brought in by the ambulance team unconscious. He has a high temperature and splenomegaly.

939. A middle aged woman is confused and dyspnoeic. Her blood pressure is high, her fundus shows retinopathy, and her urine has a high specific gravity.

940. A young man is brought into Accident and Emergency unconscious. He is pale, and sweating. His breathing is creatorus. His pupils are fixed and dilated. His reflexes' are reduced and his serum alcohol is 100 mg per 100 ml.

Theme: The Management of Abdominal Pain

Options

A. Mannitol

B. Dexamethazone

Craniotomy

D. Eye drops

E. Regular follow up

F. Interferon

G. Acyclovir

H. Primary closure

I. Laparotomy

J. Oesophageal stapling

K. Sclerotherapy

L. Tlnidazole

M. Metronidazole

N. Penicillin

Instructions

From the list of options given above choose the most approrpriate measure for each of the presentations given below. You may use each option once, more than once, or not at all.

941. A young woman who ingested three full bottles of paracetamol earlier in the day presents with fever, sweating, jaundice, and confusion. Examintion of her eyes demonstrates increasins papilloedema.

942. A middle aged man presents with an enlarged liver and feeling unwell. On physical examination you find no signs of liver disease. Investigations are normal. Liver biopsy demonstrates enlarged portal tracts and a chronic inflammatory cell infiltrate.

943. A 52-year-old man complains of chronic ill health. He presents with malaise, a low grade fever, and jaundice. His liver is large and tender, and he is jaundiced. His liver is large and tender. Biopsy of the liver demonstrates piecemeal necrosis. His HBsAg is positive and his e antigen is negative.

944. A 38-year-old man presents with blood stained vomitus. After a heavy meal in a restaurant he collapsed in the street and was brought in by the ambulance team. His condition has been stabilised, but he continues to cough up blood. He is jaundiced, and you palpate a mass in the upper right hypochondrium.

945. A middle aged man who presents in Accident a~ Emergency with acute abdominal pain. He has s~ the evening celebrating is daughters graduation

school. Over the past year he has presented into Accident and Emergency three times with a similiar complaint. Barium studies have demonstrated some smoothness of the stomach lining.

Theme: The Diagnosis of Weakness and Ill Health

Options

A. Teratoma

B. Seminoma

C. Chronic infection

D. Multiple myeloma

E. Burkitt's lymphoma

F. Non-Hodgkin's lymphoma

G. Hodgkin's disease

H. Thrombocytopenia

I. Chronic myeloid leukaemia

J. Waldenstrom's macroglobinaemia

K. Chronic lymphatic leukaemia

L. Hairy cell leukaemia

M. Acute lymphoblastic leukaemia

N. Acute myelogenous leukaemia

Instructions

From the list of options given above choose the diagnosis that most fully and accurately corresponds to the clinical details of the individual presentations given below. You may use each option once, more than once, or not at all.

946. A child is brought to you with weakness, malaise, and bone pain. On physical examination you find painfully enlarged lymph nodes and hard and enlarged testicles. He has a history of sore throats and chest infections.

947. A 51-year-old lecturer presents with lethargy, abdominal pain, fever, and weight loss. On physical examination you find a large spleen. A blood examination shows normocytic normochromic anaemia with a very high white cell count.

48. An elderly man presents with backache, pallor, and shortness of breath. He has suddenly had some difficulties with his vision. Blood examination demonstrates a high ESR, and normochromic normocytic anaemia. There is rouleux formation.

949. A young woman complains of weakness, fatigue, and anorexia. Her cervical lymph nodes are enlarged, painless, and rubbery. Her skin itches and she sometimes has night sweats. On physical examination you find her spleen and liver to be enlarged.

950. A 44-year-old man presents with ill health. He complains of wasting, fever and sweats. He does not have a skin rash, but he does have skin nodules. On physical examination you find disparate groups of lymph nodes to be enlarged.

Theme: The Diagnosis of Chest Complaints

Options

A. Anxiety
B. Myocardial infarction
C. Pulmonary embolism
D. Aortic dissection
E. Angina
F. Herpes
G. Tabes dorsalis
H. Lung infarct
 I. Pleurisy
J. Myocarditis
K. Oesophagitis
L. Peptic ulcer
M. Cholecystitis
N. Pancreatitis

Instructions

From the list of options given above choose the diagnosis that most fully accounts for the details of the individual presentations given below. You may use each option once more than once, or not at all.

951. A 40-year-old woman complains of chest pain aggr. vated by breathing. She sits up very erect and is reluctant to breath in. On examination of the chest you find clear lung fields and a tender area to the left of the sternum.

952. Following an acute streptococcal sore throat infection a middle aged man develops acute chest pain with breathlessness and pallor. His heart rate is rapid and irregular. His cardiac enzymes are normal.

953. A young woman complains of acute chest pain. It is stabbing and makes her breathless. It involves her whole chest and her lips and feet have gone numb.

954. A 52-year-old man drives himself into Accident and Emergency with an acute and stabbing chest pain. He has had the pain for more than half an hour and is in extreme distress. He is pale and sweaty and on presenting himself at the desk vomits.

955. A 33-year-old woman complains of chest pain radiating through to the back. She is overweight and decided to come in after taking a cup of hot tea which brought on her chest pain again. She says leaning forward can bring it on and that it has been getting much worse recently.

Theme: The Diagnosis of Chest Complaints

Options

A. Bronchogenic carcinoma
B. Cushing's disease
C. Hyperparathyroidism
D. Diabetes mellitus
E. Steriod abuse
F. Coaractation of the aorta
G. Conn's syndrome
H. Acromegaly
 I. Alcoholism
J. Polyarteritis nodosa
K. Systemic sclerosis
L. Idiopathic hypertension
M. Chronic pyelonephritis
   Insulinoma

Instructions

From the list of options given above choose the diagnosis that most accurately and fully captures the details of the individual presentations given below. You may use each option once, more than once, or not at all.

956. A 38-year-old woman complains of feeling bloated and recurrent chest infections. She says, she bruises very easily and has missed periods. On examination you find her blood pressure to be very high.

957. A 40-year-old man presents with sweating, headaches, and hyertension. He also complains of joint pain, muscle weakness, and numbness in both hands. Over the past few months he has become increasingly breathless and his ankles have swollen up.

958. A 48-year-old woman presents with fever, malaise, weight loss, and joint pain. She has high blood pressure and large feet. She complains of perisistent chest pain. She has a purpuric   rash and skin nodules.

959. A middle aged man presents with abdominal pain and bone pain. He has hypertension and a recent history of recurrent renal stones. His plasma calcium is high.

960. At a routine health check you carry out a fundoscopy on an apparently healthy young man. You find he has arteriolar narrowing tortuosity and an increased light reflex.

Theme: Dizziness Fits and Confusion

Options

A. Nephrotic syndrome

B. Tuberculosis

C. Intestinal hurry'

D. Recurrence of carcinoma

E. Glucose-6-phosphatase deficiency

F Pernicious anaemia

G. Nephroblastoma

H. Wilm's tumour

I. Secondaries

J. Benign postural hypotension

K. Drug interaction

L. Drug overdose

M. Chronic respiratory distress

N. Alkalosis

O. Diabetic ketoacidosis

Instructions

Choose an option from the list of diagnoses given above that accurately and fully captures the details of the presentations given below. You may use each option once, more than once, or not at all.

961. A 45-year-old man is diagnosed as having a kidney condition and treated. He soon develops postural hypotension with ankle oedema. His serum sodium is high, his potassuim normal, his urea normal, and he has heavy proteinuria.

962. A 20-year-old teacher is restless and confused. She is pale and sweaty and tachyapnoeic. Her arterial oxygen is high and her carbon dioxide is low.

963. A baby has anumber of fits, each occurring in the morning on four consecutive days. On physical examination you find the liver to be enlarged. His fasting blood sugar is low and his uric acid is high.

964. A 30-year-old salesman complains of night sweats and dizziness. His ESR is high and his blood sugar is low. He has a normocytic anaemia and sterile pyuria.

965. A 50-year-old man is brought in by his wife who says he is always fatting. He has a fresh abdominal scar. His haemoglobulin is low. His mean corpuscular volume is low. His mean corpuscular haemoglobulin concentration is low. And his glucose tolerance test shows lag storage.

Theme: ECG Interpretation

Options

A. Hypothermia

B. Pyrexia

Right atrial hypertrophy

Left atrial hypertrophy

E. Right ventricular hypertrophy

F. Left ventricular hypertrophy

G. Conduction defect

H. Myocardial infarction

I. Ischaemic heart disease

J. Pulmonary hypertension

K. Myocarditis

L. Rheumatic heart disease

M. Potassium excess

N. Hypothyroidism

Instructions

Choose an option from the above list of diagnoses that most fully and accurately corresponds to the ECG changes described below. You may use each option once, more than once, or not at all.

966. A teenage boy with dyspnoea and chest pain is brought into Accident and Emergency. He has a history of rheumatic fever. An ECG demonstrates left atrial hypertrophy and left ventricular hypertrophy. It also demonstrates waves and raised ST segment.

967. An elderly woman is found unconscious at home. An ECG demonstrates sinus bradycardia. T waves, ST depression, and flattened T waves.

968. A patient's ECG shows a biphasic P wave.

969. A patient's ECG shows T wave inversion and ST depression.

970. A 25-year-old woman complains of tiredness and malaise. Her T waves are widespread and deep.

Theme: The Diagnosis of Abdominal Pain

Options

A. Familial polyposis

B. Food poisoning

C. Anorexia-bulaemia

D. Irritable bowel syndrome

E. Crohn's disease

F. Ulcerative colitis

G. Diverticular disease

H. Gall stone ileus

I. Adhesions

J. Faecal impaction

K. Pelvic abscess

L. Rectal carcinoma

M. Colonic cancer

N. Blood dyscrasia

Instructions

From the list of options given above choose the diagnosis that fully and accurately reflects the details of the presentations given below. You may use each option once, more than once, or not at all.

971. For the past two weeks a middle aged railway engineer has complained of acute constipation. His stools are dark, but not apparently blood stained. Abdominal palpation detects a mass with moderate tenderness.

972. A 43-year-old man says he cannot finish his stool and that what he does pass is streaked with blood. He says he has always been regular. He wants to know if a laxative will help.

973. A 49-year-old lawyer complains of blood and diarrhoea. Recently she has suffered abdominal pain, fever, and general ill health. On palpation you find tenderness in the lower abdomen.

974. A young woman presents with recurrent abdominal pain, episodic diarrhoea, malaise, and fever. Over the past few years she has felt her health to be declining. At presentation she complains of severe abdominal pain and constipation.

975. A young woman complains of cramp like abdominal pain, and difficulties with bowel movements. Acute abdominal pain is frequently relieved by embarrassing flatulence. Barium studies and sigmoidoscopy have proved inconclusive.

Theme: The Diagnosis of Painful Intercourse

Options

A. Genital herpes
B. Human papilloma virus
C. Chancroid
D. *Candida albicans*
E. *Chlamydial trachomatis*
F. Prostatis
G. Syphilis
H. *Eschiera coli*
I. Mulloscum contagiosum
J. *Haemophilus ducreyi*
K. Donovania
L. Gardnerella
M. Gonorrhoea
N. Granuloma inguinale

Instructions

From the list of options given above choose the diagnosis that accurately captures the details of the individual presentations given below. You may use each option once, more than once, or not at all.

976. A young woman complains of pain during intercourse. She has a mild vaginal discharge and a burning sensation when passing urine.

977. A 28-year-old woman says she finds intercourse painful. She has a vaginal discharge which is very foul smelling.

978. A 33-year-old woman says she must leave off with intercourse because of intense pain. She has a fever, headache, and is generally unwell. On examination you find inguinal lymphadenopathy and small painful genital ulcers.

979. A 45-year-old man presents with pain during intercourse. He says the pain is sharp and stabbing and from the tip of the penis. He also complains of a pelvic ache and a burning sensation.

980. A young woman complains of painful intercourse. There is a mild degree of vaginal pain within the

pelvis and worse with penetration. There are no other symptoms or signs.

Theme: The Diagnosis of High Fever and Coughing

Options

A. Listeria monocytogenes
B. Strychine poisoning
C. Mushroom poisoning
D. Rabies
E. Entericfever
F. Shigella
G Dental abscess
H. Erysipelas
I. Bordetalla pertusis
J. Tetanus
K. Coryza
L. Bronchiectasis
M. Influenzae
N. Meningitis

Instructions

From the list of options given above choose the most likely diagnosis given the clinical details of each case presented below. Each option may be used once, more than once, or not at all.

981. A child has a cough and a fever. During the day, and especially at night, he has fits of coughing, and cannot help himself. His inspirations are harsh. At first his mother thought he had a cold, but he has not got better.

982. A healthy young woman who likes grow in vegetables, raising animals, and preparing food complains of fever and aches and pains. She also has a sore throat, conjunctivitis, and diarrhoea.

983. A young woman recently returned from holiday in Kenya presents with a severe headache and fever. He also complains of anorexia, abdominal pain, and

constipation. On physical examination you find multiple, small, and raised pink spots on his chest.

984. A child with abdominal pain and bloody diarrhoea is brought in by her parents. The child has a fever, headache, and some neck stiffness. The CSF is sterile. The mother says a number of children at her daughter's school are similarly ill.

985. A young farmer presents with facial spasms and difficulty closing his mouth. For the past week he has had fever, malaise, and headache. A month earlier he had been involved in a tractor accident.

Theme: The Diagnosis of Abdominal Pain

Options

A. Gastric ulcer
B. Gastric atrophy
C. Non-ulcer dyspepsia
D. Basal pneumonia
E. Retrocaecal appendicitis
F. *Helicobacter pylori*
G. Duodenitis
H. Carcinoma of the stomach
I. Oesophagitis
J. Hepatitis
K. Acute pancreatitis
L. Duodenal peptic ulcer
M. Acute cholecystitis
N. Myocardial infarction

Instructions

From the list above choose the option that most accurately and fully reflects the details of the individual presentations given below. Each option may be used once, more than once, or not at all.

986. A 32-year-old man points to an area of acute epigastric pain with his right index finger. The pain is worse at night and is relieved by taking food. It is also reliev by taking antacids. His serum amylase is slig elevated

987. A 48-year-old short order cook presents with nausea and acute abdominal pain boring through to the back. The epigastrium is very tender. He has had three similiar bouts in the past 18 months. A barium meal is normal.

988. A 51-year-old woman complains of chronic abdominal pain around the umbilicus. She often suffers from indigestion, abdominal pain, and vomiting. She had a thyroidectomy 12 years ago and is on a replacement regime. A barium meal shows an absence of mucosal folds.

989. A 39-year-old marketing executive presents with acute epigastric pain. The pain is continuous and it has been increasing in intensity over the past day and a half. It radiates to the right hypochondrium

990. A middle aged man presents with acute abdominal pain that radiates through to the back. The pain is severe and causes him to feel sick and vomit repeatedly. On physical examination you find the abdomen to be tender. His serum amylase is 5 times greater than normal.

Theme: ECG Interpretation

Options

A. Digoxin toxicity

B. Myocarditis

C. Dextrocardia

D. Wolf-Parkinson-White Syndrome

E. Ventricularaneurysm

F. Valve defect

G. Recent myocardial infarction

H. Hypothyroidism

I. Complete heart block

J. Hypertension

K. Hypokalaemia

Hyperkalaemia

Sick sinus syndrome

Pericarditis

Instructions

From the list of options given above choose the most likely diagnosis for the ECG abnormalities described below. Each option may be used once, more than once, or not at all.

991. An 80-year-old woman suffers repeated drop attacks. An ECG reveals left ventricular hypertrophy, left axis deviation, atrial ectopics, and atrial tachycardia.

992. An elderly man is tired and nauseous. On examination of his ECG traces you find deep Q waves, an elevated ST segment, and T wave inversion.

993. A 56-year-old woman is drowsy and confused. Her ECG findings are a profound bradycardia, absent P waves, Q waves, tall T waves, and a long QT interval.

994. A 65-year-old man has an irregular pulse. His ECG shows a sawtooth pattern. The QRS complexes are irregularly spaced.

995. A patient's ECG shows bradycardia, a prolonged PR interval, and ventricular ectopics.

Theme: The Clinical Diagnosis of Common Infections

Options

A. Influenzae

B. Hepatitis

C. Meningitis

D. Coryza

E. Diptheria

F. Rubella

G. Mononucleosis

H. Candidiasis

I. Poliomyelitis

J. Tuberculosis

K. Brucellosis

L. Staphylococcus

M. Streptococcus

N. Herpes

Instructions

Choose a diagnosis from the list of options given above that is most likely to apply to the individual presentations given below. You may use each option once, more than once, or not at all.

996. An elderly man presents with a sore throat and complains of losing his voice. Examination of the throat finds the oral cavity erythematous and sporadically covered with white and yellow patches. He is apparently healthy otherwise.

997. A young farmer complains of a high fever and drenching sweats lasting two or three days. He has had a severe headache, backache and felt very depressed. He says he has had three similar episodes in the past month.

998. A 23-year-old student presents with weakness, malaise, fever, and yellow sclerae. Her upper right abdomen is very tender, and her joints ache.

999. A teenager has a terrible headache and a skin rash on the face. His cervical lymph nodes are enlarged. After admission the rash involves his chest and upper arms. He says his joints are very painful, especially his knees.

1000. An immigrant child is brought to you with a sore throat and fever. His breathing is laboured and his voice is deep. The trachea is covered with a thin membrane. His cervical lymph nodes are enlarged.

Theme: The Diagnosis of Feel Unwell

Options

A. Hepatitis A
B. Hepatitis B
C. Hepatitis C
D. Gall stones
E. Pancreatitis
F. Cholangeosclerosis
G. HIV infection
H. Cirrhosis
I. Chronic persistent hepatitis

J. Chronic active hepatitis

K. Secondaries

L. Hepatocellular carcinoma

M. Leukaemia

N. Lymphoma

Instructions

From the list of options given above choose a diagnosis that accurately and fully corresponds to the details of the individual presentations given below. Each option may be used once, more than once, or not at all.

1001. An elderly man presents with severe epigastric pain radiating to the right hypochondrium. The pain has been worsening over tne past day and a half and goes through to his back and shoulders. The patient feels sick and has vomited several times. He is jaundiced.

1002. A middle aged man complains of his appearance. His wife says his eyes are yellow. On physical examination you find mild hepatomegaly. His alkaline phosphatase, albumin, and globulin are normal. He says he is a teetotaller.

1003. A healthy young waiter complains of feeling unwell with nausea, vomiting, and diarrhoea. He has a headache, fever, and abdominal pain. On palpation you find the liver to be tender and enlarged.

1004. A 34-year-old stockbroker presents with jaundice and physical exhaustion. His liver and spleen are enlarged and you notice he has spider naevi on both cheeks. He says he is a moderate drinker and that he has been unwell for more than a year.

1005. A middle aged social worker presents with abdominal pain and fever. She has been unwell for two weeks and feels she is getting worse rather than better. Her urine is dark and her stools are pale. She has tender lymph nodes and joint pain.

Theme: The Diagnosis of Abnormal Chest X-rays

Options

A. Sarcoidosis
B. Histiocytosis
C. *Aspergillus fumigattus*
D. Idiopathic thrombocytopenia
E. Polyarteritis nodosa
F. Hyperparathyroidism
G. Silent infarction
H. Asthma
I. Emphysema
J. Lung fibrosis
K Pleurisy
L. Lung collapse
M. Tuberculosis
N. Lung problem

Instructions

From the list of options given above choose the diagnosis that most accurately and fully reflects the details of the individual presentations given below. You may use each option once, more than once, or not at all.

1006. A young woman complains of sore eyes, a dull chest pain, malaise, and a low grade fever. She thinks she has had a recurrent low grade fever for four months. A chest X-ray shows bilateral hilar enlargement.

1007. A middle aged pharmaceutical engineer presents with increasing breathlessness and cough. He doesn't smoke. On chest X-ray you find diffuse bilatral mottling and multiple small cystic lesions. Six months ago he had a pneumothorax.

1008. For the past three years a young man has complained of recurrent bouts of pneumonia with wheeziness, cough, fever, and malaise. His sputum is tenacious. Peripheral blood shows a very high ESR and IgE.

1009. A 30-year-old computer engineer with a long history of asthma and rhinitis presents with wheezing, cough and fever. A chest X-ray shows patchy consolidation. Physical examination shows multiple tender subcutaneous nodules and purpura.

1010. A 43-year-old man presents with chest pain and a cough. He complains of a fullness and pressure in the chest and a sharp pain affecting two or three ribs on the right side. A chest X-ray shows right sided hilar enlargement.

Theme: The Diagnosis of Abnormal Bleeding

Options

A. Haemolytic uraemic syndrome

B. Dessiminated malignancy

C. Dessiminated intravascular coagulation

D. Systemic lupus erythematosis

E. Idiopathic thrombocytopenic purpura

F. Von Willebrand's disease

G. Transfusion reaction

H. Chronic lymphatic leukaemia

I. Haemophilia A

J. Drug reaction

K. Viral infection

L. Vitamin K deficiency

M. Cholestatic jaundice

N. Hormonal imbalance

Instructions

From the list of options given above choose the diagnosis that most fully and accurately captures the presentations set out below. You may use each option once, more than once, or not at all,

1011. A 51-year-old woman with a history of jaundice presents with gross haematuria. On physical examination you find bruises of various ages, especially on the lower legs. Her prothrombin time is elevated.

1012. A 24-year-old builder accidentally drives a nail through his foot. He cleans the wound himself with antiseptic solution, but develops a high fever afterwards. A few days later he begins to bleed from his mouth and nose.

1013. A middle aged woman complains of easy bruising, purpura and heavy periods. She frequently has nose bleeds. Her spleen is not enlarged. Her platelet autoantibodies are negative.

1014. A healthy young man is involved in a cycling accident and makes a very poor recovery with heavy bleeding into his calf muscles. His prothrombin times and bleeding times are normal.

1015. A young woman complains of very heavy bleeding and bruising. While playing tennis she injures her knee and suffers haemoarthrosis. Investigation shows her bleeding time to be prolonged.

Theme: The Diagnosis of Confusion

Options

A. Viral encephalitis
B. Brain primary
C. Epilepsy
D. Cerebrovascular accident
E. Pancreatic tumour
F. Diabetic ketoacidosis
G. Psychiatric illness
H. Influenzae
I. Subarachnoid haemorrhage
J. Nephroma
K. Acute intermittent porphyria
L. Variegate porphyria
M. Liver failure
N. Amyloidosis

Instructions

From the list of options given above choose the diagnosis that most fully and accurately corresponds to the individual presentations given below. You may use an option once, more than once, or not at all.

1016. A young woman complains of sweating, palpitations, abdominal pain, and weakness. On bringing herself into Accident and Emergency she is aggressive and confused. She has a seizure and falls unconscious. Her serum insulin is high.

1017. A 27-year-old PhD student presents with abdominal pain, nausea, and vomiting. His breathing is rapid and shallow. He is confused. On examination you find the breath sweet smelling, the eyes sunken, and the body temperature below normal.

1018. A 26-year-old woman presents with abdominal pain, vomiting, and constipation. She also complains of numbness and clumsiness in her legs. She has been very depressed and anxious. Her urine is dark.

1019. An elderly man with a history of rheumatoid arthritis presents with abdominal pain, a swollen face, and swollen eyelids. His JVP is normal and his urine is frothy. Urine examination shows paraproteinaemia.

1020. A student who has ingested three full bottle of paracetamol is brought in with acute abdominal pain. She is very angry and confused. She vomits several times and falls unconscious.

Theme: Investigating a Change of Bowel Habits

Options

A. Erythrocyte sedimentation rate

B. Stool culture

C. Per rectum examination

D. Full blood count

E. Haemoglobulin

F. Plain abdominal X-ray

G. Proctoscopy

H. Sigmoidoscopy

I. Abdominal palpation

J. Barium enema

K. Laparotomy

L. Double enema test

M. White blood cell count

N. Stool examination

Instructions

How would you investigate further the following cases of a change of bowel habits? Choose the single most telling and appropriate investigation from the list of options given above. You may use each option once, more than once, or not at all.

1021. A teenager complains of acute abdominal pain. He has felt unwell and unable to pass stools since a game of football yesterday afternoon. On physical examination you find a tense, smooth and tender lower abdominal swelling.

1022. A 55-year-old man complains of constipation and colicky abdominal pain. On physical examination you find a palpable and mobile abdominal mass. The patient appears very pale.

1023. A young adult complains of recurrent attacks of diarrhoea. She says her stools contain blood and mucous. Sometimes she has a low grade fever.

1024. A 42-year-old train driver complains of diarrhoea. He says he has always been regular. He says his stools contain blood and that he passes mucous first thing in the morning.

1025. An elderly woman cannot pass stools. She is bedridden and incontinent. She has taken laxatives and they did give her some relief, but she still feels very constipated.

Theme: Appropriate Investigations in Chronic Fatigue

Options

A. Chromosomal analysis

B. Full blood count

C. Blood film

D. Barium meal

E. Sternal marrow biopsy

F. Gastroscopy

G. Abdominal X-ray

H. Fractional test meal

 I. Serum B12

 J. Stool examination

K. Haemoglobulin estimation

 L. Liver function tests

M. Lymphangiogram

N. Lymph node biopsy

Instructions

Examine the following cases and choose that investigation from the list of options given above that best corresponds to the most telling and appropriate initial investigation you would order. Each option may be used once, more than once, or not at all.

1026. A 46-year-old lecturer complains of being chronically tired. She says that her two-year-old is just too much for her, and that she and her husband have trouble getting him to accept a vegetarian diet. On physical examination you find the patient to be pale and off colour.

1027. A 28-year-old programmer complains of fatigue and intermittent fevers. On physical examination you find him to have swollen lymph nodes and upper left sided abdominal distension. He has a high E.S.R.

1028. A 63-year-old man complains of tiredness and indigestion. He has been treated with antacids six weeks previously and the treatment has helped but the pains in his abdomen have returned and become more or less constant.

1029. A 48-year-old man complains of tiredness and abdominal pain. He says his gums bleed when he brushes his teeth. On physical examination you find an enlarged spleen and bruises of various ages.

1030. A 53-year-old physical education instructor complains of malaise, fatigue, a sore tongue, and diarrhoea. On physical examination you find some atrophy of the tongue, and a very high pulse rate.

Theme: The Diagnosis of Substernal Chest Pain

Options

A. Atrial fibrillation
B. Angina pectoris
C. Reflux oesophagitis
D. Peptic ulcer
E. Oesophageal carcinoma
F. Asthma
G. Bornholm's disease
H. Myocardial infarction
 I. Pulomonary tuberculosis
 J. Pneumonia
K. Spontaneous pneumothorax
L. Dissecting aneurysm
M. Pulmonary embolism
N. Pleurisy

Instructions

All of these patients complain of chest pain. Choose a diagnosis from the options listed above that most accurately and fully reflects their more specific complaints. You may use an option once, more than once, or not at all.

1031. A middle aged women with sedentary habits has chest pain aggravated by breathing and coughing. She has a slight fever. Two months ago she had pneumonia but recovered fully.

1032. A short overweight middled aged woman com-plains of chest pain below her sternum. The pain is worse at night and always starts up after meals. She has had five children.

1033. A 48-year-old man presents with acute chest pain in the substernal area. The pain radiates to his neck and arm. He says that the pain also goes through to his back.

1034. A 62-year-old housewife complains of central chest pain after a heavy meal. The pain goes to her neck, she says, and her finger tips on her left hand are numb. Her serum transaminase and lactic dehydro-genase are normal.

1035. A young asthmatic comes to you with chest pain of sudden onset. The pain is on the lower left side. He says the pain followed a bout of coughing and has left him breathless.

Theme: The Diagnosis of Haematuria

Options

A. Anticoagulant therapy
B. Bladder tumour
C. Pregnancy
D. Inflammatory bowel disease
E. Wilm's tumour
F. Renal calculi
G. Acute glomerulonephritis
H. Angioneurotic oedema
I. Cystitis
J. Prostatic enlargement
K. Chronic pyelonephritis
L. Papilloma
M. Carcinoma of the kidney
N. Urethral caruncle

Instructions

Examine the following five cases of dark urine and decide which of the above mentioned diagnoses is most likely given the somewhat limited information you have before you. You may use each diagnosis once, more than once, or not at all.

1036. A 12-year-old boy has had a sore throat for the past month with headache, malaise, and a persistent low grade fever. You notice some fullness in the face and very dark urine.

1037. A 41-year-old roan complains of recurrent abdominal pains, especially on the left side. He says the pain travels down to his scrotum. And he says his urine has been dark for months.

1038. A fifty-year-old diabetic complains of feeling unwell, frequency, dysuria, and dark urine. Over the past 3 months he has felt feverish.

1039. A 32-year-old woman complains of sudden frequency, nocturia, and vomiting. She does not have a fever and she has missed a period. Her urine is dark.

1040. A 62-year-old woman complains of feeling unwell and weight loss. She looks pale and unwell and on palpation you discover a mass in her left flank. She has had painless haematuria for three months.

Theme: The Diagnosis of Abdominal Pain

Options

A. Peritonitis
B. Gall stones
C. Crohn's disease
D. Gall stones
E. Duodenal ulcer
F. Hiatus hernia
G. Reflux oesophagitis
H. Carcinoma of the head of the pancreas
I. Carcinoma of the tail of the pancreas
J. Acute pancreatitis
K. Chronic pancreatitis
L. Gastric ulcer
M. Oesophageal tear
N. Helicobacter pylori infection

Instructions

From the list of options given above choose the most likely diagnosis for the presentations given below. You may use each option once, more than once, or not at all.

1041. An elderly man presents with abdominal pain, anorexia, and weight loss. The pain is dull and penetrating through to the back. It helps him with the pain to stoop forwards. His right leg is inflamed and tender.

1042. A middle aged man complains of persistent abdoimnal pain. He says antacids and food help him with the pain but that it will not go away. Sometimes

he feels sick and vomits and that helps. Recently he
has lost his appetite and weight.

1043. An elderly woman presents with painless jaundice
and weight loss. On physical examination you find
the gall bladder to be enlarged. She enjoys smoking
and drinking.

1044. A middle aged man presents with acute abdominal
pain in the epigastrium. The pain radiates to the
back between the scapulae. It is excruciating. The
patient is nauseous and vomits repeatedly.

1045. A 38-year-old man complains of recurrent bouts of
abdominal pain. The pain begins below the sternum
and moves through to the back. Sometimes the pain
is disabling and the patient cannot leave his bed.
When he has the pain he loses his appetite completely and has lost as much as a stone in weight.

Theme: Headache

Options

A. CT scan of head

B. EEG

C. ECG

D. Lumbar puncture

E. X-ray skull

F. Angiography

G. Fundus examination

H. Intubation and ventilation

I. Nasal catheter oxygen

J. Psychiatric analysis

K. ESR estimation

L. Aspirin

Instructions

For each numbered item below, select the most appropriate
answer from the options listed above. Each option may be
selected once, more than once or not at all.

1046. A 12-year-old boy is recovering from his bilater
parotitis. He develops headache and delirium.

1047. A 42-year man develops headache, transient vision loss and lost consciousness. All his symptoms subside within 2 hours.

1048. A 47-year-old man complains of sudden severe headache in the occiput.

1049. A 52-year-old man presents with headache, pinpoint pupil and deep slow respiration of 6/min.

1050. A 48-year-old female complains of continuous severe headache pressing her head like a band.

1051. A 46-year-old man has severe headache and red eye. His fundoscopy reveals pale disc.

1052. A 69-year-old female present with headache that is more marked while she is combing her hair. She also has shoulder and hip musde weakness.

Theme: Pain Management in Labour

Options

A. General anaesthesia

B. Spinal anaesthesia

C. Epidural anaesthesia

D. Pudental block

E. Entonox

F. IM morphine

G. IV Pethidine

H. NSAID

I. Paracetamol

J. Prochlorperazine

K. Transcutaneous nerve stimulation

L. Pressure massage

M. Acupuncture

Instructions

For each numbered item below, select the most appropriate answer from the options listed above. Each option may be elected once, more than once or not at all.

53. 28-year-old primi delivered a baby 30 minutes ago and she is still bleeding vaginally. The decision to remove the placenta manually was made.

1054. A 32-year-old female has prolonged labour. Cervix is 8 cm dilated in 12 hours. She said that the contractions are more painful and she could no longer tolerate it.

1055. A pregnant mother discusses about pain relief in the antenatal clinic. She insists upon her freedom of movement during her labour and she wants to walk during labour.

1056. 29-year-old primi is in labour. Cervix is 9 cm dilated and the head is in occipito posterior position.

1057. A 32-year-old gravida 2 complains of pain during uterine contractions. Cervix is 6 cm dilated. She already received 2 injections of pethidine.

Theme: Vaginal Discharge Diagnosis

Options

A. Candidiasis
B. *Trichomonas vaginalis*
C. Bacterial vaginosis
D. Carcinoma vulva
E. Gonococcal PID
F. Chlamydial PID
G. Herpes simplex
H. Granuloma inguinale
I. Tuberculosis
J. Syphilis
K. Eczema

Instructions

For each numbered item below, select the most appropriate answer from the options listed above. Each option may be selected once, more than once or not at all.

1058. A 25-year-old female complains of thick white vaginal discharge. Vaginal pH is 4. Vaginal smear shows numerous mycelia.

1059. A 32-year-old female complains of foul smelling vaginal discharge. On smear, clue cells and squamous cells are present.

1060. A 22-year-old sexually active female complains of vaginal discharge and deep dysparaunia. Smear for Gonococcus is negative.

1061. A 31-year-old sexually active female has thin vaginal discharge and pain during micturation. On examination she had multiple ulcers at the vaginal introitus.

Theme: Chest Pain

Options

A. Exercise ECG

B. Admit to cardiac intensive care unit and start on O_2 and morphine

C. NSAID

D. Paracetamol

E. Diazepam

F. Continuous pH monitoring

G. Gastroscopy

H. No treatment

I. Take patient to operating the threatres·

Instructions

For each numbered item below, select me most appropriate answer from the options listed above. Each option may be selected once, more than once or not at all.

1062. A 55-year-old male presents with sudden severe chest pain penetrating through the chest wall to back. His BP is 180/110 mm Hg.

1063. A 48-year-old obese female complains of central chest pain, which is worse on lying or bending forwards. She also complains of sour taste in the mouth in the morning.

1064. A 58-year-old patient with family history of ischaemic heart disease presents with central chest pain. The pain is variably related to exercise.

1065. A 62-year-old chronic smoker presents with dull central chest pain. His BP is 110/70 mm Hg, pulse 110/min. ECG shows ST segment elevation and Q waves in leads II, III and avF.

1066. A 42-year-old male presents with sharp central chest pain, which is relieved by leaning forward and worse on lying. Most of the ECG leads show ST elevation.

Theme: Fever and Rash in Children

Options

A. Meningococcus
B. Ebstein barr virus
C. HIV
D. Herpes simplex
E. Erythema toxicum
F. Roseola infantum
G. Kawasaki disease
H. Encephalitis
I. Henoch schonlein purpura
J. Idiopathic thrombocytopenic purpura
K. Porphyria cutanea tarda
L. Malaria
M. Measles

Instructions

For each numbered item below, select the most appropriate answer from the options listed above. Each option may be selected once, more than once or not at all.

1067. A 14-year-old girl developed sore throat, fever and spleenomegaly and was started on ampicillin. On the third day she developed rashes all over the body.

1068. A 2-year-old boy presents with high fever, Erythema and peeling of skin over palms and soles. On examination there is maculo papular rash all over the body and lymphadenopathy is present.

1069. A 2-year-old child develops high fever, febrile fits and was treated with paracetamol syrup. Fever subsides and the child discharged. Two days later he develops florid rash throughout the body. The baby is alert and well.

1070. A 6-year-old boy developed mild fever and malaise. On examination he had multiple perioral and labial ulcers and rashes.

1071. A 5-year-old child was sent from school since she developed high fever and headache. The teacher noted multiple non-blanching rashes.

Theme: Genetic Disorders Mode of Inheritance

Options

A. Autosomal dominance
B. Autosomal codominance
C. Autosomal recessive
D. X-linked
E. Polygenic
F. Single gene defect

Instructions

For each numbered item below, select the most appropriate answer from the options listed above. Each option may be selected once, more than once or not at all.

1072. A 1-year-old male child presents with failure to thrive and anaemia. His father has had a work up for anaemia and his mother received multiple transfusion of blood.

1073. A 28-year-old man presents with increasing instability, ataxia and tremor. His father and his grand father had the same disease and died at there 40's.

1074. A 5-year-old boy developed swelling of his left knee with trivial injury. He had similar episodes like this before. His maternal uncle and his grand father had same complaints.

1075. An 18-year-old female underwent caries tooth extraction and developed profuse bleeding. On history she revealed menorrhagia. Her mother and her grand father had the same disease.

1076. A 21-year-old female developed insulin dependent diabetes mellitus. Her uncle and grandmother had the same disease.

Theme: Sudden Loss of Vision

Options

A. Central retinal artery occlusion
B. Central retinal vein occlusion
C. Retinal detachment
D. Uveitis
E. Acute glaucoma
F. Occipital infarct
G. Pituitary infarct
H. Migraine
I. Chorio retinitis
J. Cataract
K. Optic neuitis
L. Cranial arteritis

Instructions

For each numbered item below, select the most appropriate answer from the options listed above. Each option may be selected once, more than once or not at all.

1077. A 40-year-old male presents with sudden loss of vision, vomiting and red eye for 1 day.

1078. A 23-year-old male complains of detoriating vision. In the past he had several attacks of backpain.

1079. A 64-year-old patient with a long history of hypertension and diabetes, woke up in the morning with sudden loss of sight in his left eye.

1080. A 68-year-old female with lung cancer and cough was admitted to the hospital. The next morning she couldn't see her breakfast tray.

1081. A 62-year-old female developed transient loss of vision. She also has headache, malaise and proximal muscle weakness.

Theme: Earache

Options

A. Acute otitis media
B. Chronic otitis media
C. Otitis externa
D. Presbyacusis
E. Tempero mandibular joint dysfunction
F. Herpes zoster
G. Ear drum perforation
H. Vestibular neuronitis
I. Acute tonsillitis
J. Trigeminal neuralgia
K. Dental caries

Instructions

For each numbered item below, select the most appropriate answer from the options listed above. Each option may be selected once, more than once or not at all.

1082. A 4-year-old child develops upper respiratory tract infection. Her mother treats this illness with paracetamol syrup. On the fourth day, the baby develops ear pain and didn't allow her mother to touch the ear.

1083. A 25-year-old male went for a holiday. After 7 days of swimming, he developed pain in both his ears.

1084. A 54-year-old female develops mild fever, malaise and ear pain. 3 days later she developed multiple painful vesicles over her ear canal and external auditory meatus.

1085. A 23-year-old lady develops pain and discharge in her right ear. 2 weeks ago she had treatment for wax. At the time of the procedure of syringing she developed acute pain.

1086. A 48-year-old female complains of left ear pain, which is worse on swallowing. Her husband noted nocturnal bruxism.

Theme: Anticoagulation

Options

A. Subcutaneous heparin 5000 u twice daily

B. Intravenous heparin

C. Intravenous dextran

D. Oral warfarin

E. Vitamin K

F. Crepe bandage

G. Graduated compression bandage

H. Leg massage

I. Radiograph of leg

J. None required

K. Aspirin

Instructions

For each numbered item below, select the most appropriate answer from the options listed above. Each option may be selected once, more than once or not at all.

1087. A 45-year-old obese man is going to undergo bilateral varicose vein surgery.

1088. A 60-year-old patient underwent total hip replacement. 2 weeks ago and develops deep vein thrombosis.

1089. A 35-year fit man is planned to have hernia repair as a day case surgery.

1090. A 48-year-old man seeks advice regarding his air travel that extends for about 18 hours. His father died at the age of 58 due to pulmonary embolism.

1091. A 75-year-old frail man develops pneumonia.

Theme: Varicose Vein Treatment

Options

A. Sclerotherapy

B. Varicose vein surgery

C. Heparin

D. Crepe bandage

E. Graduated compression stocking

F. Weight reduction

G. Doppler scan

H. Embolectomy

I. Laproscopy

J. Skin grafting

K. Leg elevation alone

Instructions

For each numbered item below, select the most appropriate answer from the options listed above. Each option may be selected once, more than once or not at all.

1092. A 46-year-old female with a body mass index of 27 presents with bilateral varicose veins.

1093. A 36-year-old smoker with a body mass index of 33 presents with severe varicose veins in the right leg. On examination she had mild varicosity in the left leg also.

1094. A 47-year-old man has bilateral varicose veins and eczematous changes in both the lower limbs around the ankle but there is no ulceration.

1095. A 38-year-old female presents with severe bilateral varicosity. She already had two varicose surgery in the past 3 years.

1096. A 45-year-old man presents with varicosity and swelling of the left leg. 2 years ago he had deep vein thrombosis of left leg and from that time onwards, the swelling persists.

Theme: Preventive Medicine

Options

A. Benzyl penicillin lM

B. Acyclovir

C. Reassurance

D. Notification to communicable disease control office

E. Serum antibody titre

F. Quarantine

G. Prophylaxis for contacts

H. Immunization for contacts

I. Barrier nursing

Instructions

For each numbered item below, select the most appropriate answer from the options listed above. Each option may be selected once, more than once or not at all.

1097. A 23-year-old female on her 2nd trimester presents with mild fever and rashes throughout her body, which she contracted from her 3-year-old niece.

1098. A mother rang you and very much worried because her son's best friend develops viral meningitis and was admitted in hospital.

1099. A 15-year-old healthy boy complains of recurrent sore throat from his childhood.

1100. A 5-year-old boy returned from his uncle's house in Calcutta developed diarrhoea. His uncle owns a restaurant there.

1101. A 8-year-old boy develops fever and headache. For the past few hours he is drowsy with altered consciousness.

1102. A family physician examining a febrile child with headache and rashes asks you in phone about the next action.

1103. A 10-Year-old boy is returning home after a successful renal transplant. In home his younger brother is having chicken pox.

Theme: Breast Lump-Next Step

Options

A. Eliciting a family history

B. Triple assessment strategy

C. CT scan

D. FNAC

E. Stereotactic needle biopsy

F. Stereotactic core biopsy

G. Wide local excision

H. Ultrasound

I. Mammography

Instructions

For each numbered item below, select the most appropriate answer from the options listed above. Each option may be selected once, more than once or not at all.

1104. A 27-year-old female is having a lump of 2 cm size in the upper and outer quadrant it is freely mobile, firm in consistency. She is having needle phobias.

1105. A 26-year-old female complains of bilateral lumpiness and pain that is more marked just before menstruation.

1106. A 41-year-old female presents with a 3 cm mass fixed to the skin. There are no palpable nodes in the axilla.

1107. A 52-year-old female on routine mammography shows a suspicious area with micro calcification. On clinical examination there is no palpable mass.

Theme: Abdominal Pain–Next Investigation

Options

A. Gastroscopy

B. ERCP

C. Oral cholecystography

D. Abdominal X-ray

E. IVU

F. Ultrasound abdomen

G. Blood glucose

H. Laproscopy

I. Urine porphyrins

J. Echocardiogram

K. Chest X-ray

Instructions

For each numbered item below, select the most appropriate answer from the options listed above. Each option may be selected once, more than once or not at all.

1108. A 62-year-old man presents with perspiration and dizziness. His BP is 100/70 mm Hg and he complains of abdominal and back pain. On examination, aortic pulsation is more prominent.

1109. A 65-year-old alcoholic presents with recurrent abdominal pain, which is relieved by leaning forward.

1110. A 46-year-old obese female complains of recurrent pain under her right lower ribs after eating fatty foods.

1111. A 48-year-old patient presents with history of recurrent epigastric pain on lying position. Now his pain becomes constant.

1112. A 16-year-old boy complains of right lower abdominal pain, which was initially around umbilicus. He then develops increased frequency of micturation.

Theme: Diagnosis of Testicular Pain

Options

A. Torsion testis

B. Epidimitis

C. Tubercular of chitis

D. Tumor

E. Trauma

F. Hydrocele

G. Syphilis

H. Varicocele

Instructions

For each numbered item below, select the most appropriate answer from the options listed above. Each option may be selected once, more than once or not at all.

1113. 16-year-old boy complains of severe left testicular pain while riding bicycle

1114. A 38-year-old man develops testicular pain, which is more, marked after prolonged standing.

1115. A 26-year-old man developed testicular pain, which diminishes in intensity when the testis is lifted up.

1116. A 30-year-old man developed testicular swelling for about 3 months. Then he developed a peculiar ache in the swelling.

1117. A 36-year-old immigrant with low-grade fever and night sweats presents with mild testicular pain. He also has backache.

Theme: Diagnosis of Lower Intestinal Disorders

Options

A. Ulcerative proctatis
B. Ulcerative pancolitis
C. Crohn's disease
D. Diverticulitis
E. Tuberculosis
F. Glandular carcinoma
G. Amoebiasis
H. Typhoid colitis
I. Sigmoid carcinoma
J. Angiodysplasia
K. lschaemic colitis
L. Sigmoid volvulus
M. Pseudomembranous colitis

Instructions

For each numbered item below, select the most appropriate answer from the options listed above. Each option may be selected once, more than once or not at all.

1118. A 62-year-old man developed crampy abdominal pain, which is relieved by passing stools for the past 4 months. Stools are watery and mixed with blood. Sigmoidoscopy reveals stricture with bleeding.

1119. A 24-year-old man developed sore throat and was treated with ampicillin. 8 days after the start of the treatment he developed bloody diarrhoea. Sigmoidoscopy shows white exudates attached to the colonic wall.

1120. A 24-year-old female present with complains of bloody diarrhoea for 2 months. On examination anal fissures present. Sigmoidoscopy shows patchy aphthous like ulcers in the transverse and descending colon.

1121. A 32-year-old man presents with alternating bloody diarrhoea and constipation for 1 month. Sigmoidoscopy reveals continuous granular appearance of the lower 13 cm of the sigmoid colon.

1122. A 62-year-old man presents with weight loss, malaise and easy fatigability. His Hb is 8 mg/dl and MCV is 68-fl. barium enema didn't enter the ascending colon.

1123. A 48-year-old immigrant complains of low grade fever, night chills and vague right iliac fossa mass. He was treated as regional ileitis and the symptoms didn't subside.

Theme: Urinary Tract Symptoms–Investigation

Options

A. Stain for acid fast bacilli

B. IVU

C. Radio nuclide scan

D. Urine culture

E. Urine for RBC casts

F. Cystoscopy

G. Micturating cystourethrography

H. KUB Radiograph

I. Ultrasound

J. Urine flow studies

Instructions

For each numbered item below, select the most appropriate answer from the options listed above. Each option may be selected once, more than once or not at all.

1124. A 1-year-old child developed fever and *E. coli* was cultured and treated. 1 month later the child is well and in good health.

1125. A 33-year-old female develops signs of urinary tract infection and on culture Proteus was identified.

1126. A 21-year-old asymtomatic man passed red urine. Microscopy shows numerous red cells.

1127. A 6-year-old chronically ill girl develops fever, jaundice. Urinalysis reveals numerous RBC and WBCs.

1128. A 16-year-old boy presents with low grade fever and weight loss. Urine shows numerous pus cells but no organism was identified on routine culture.

1129. A 28-year-old man presents with severe pain radiating from back to groin. Urine examination shows few RBCs.

Theme: Weight Loss

Options

A. Anorexia nervosa

B. Cardiac cachexia

C. Starvation

D. Thyrotoxicosis

E. Giardiasis

F. Carcinoma lung

G. Tuberculosis

H. Depression

I. Achalasia cardia

J. HIV

K. Cryptomenorrhoea

Instructions

For each numbered item below, select the most appropriate answer from the options listed above. Each option may be selected once, more than once or not at all.

1130. A 68-year-old man lost about 5 kg over the past 3 months. He also complains of diarrhoea and palpitations. ECG shows absent 'a ' waves but ST segment is normal.

1131. A 18-year-old female student was brought by her mother with history of 8 kg weight loss and 4 months amenorrhoea. But she says she is healthy and denies her weight loss.

1132. A 34-year-old businessman lost about 3 kg in the past 2 months. He told that he had started a new construction work 3 months ago. He denies stress but complains of easy fatigability.

1133. A 60-year-old man with more than 40 years history of smoking presents with 5 kg weight loss over the past 3 months.

1134. A 40-year immigrant man with chronic fever and weight loss. Though the exact weight lost is not known, his shirt is obviously hanging loosely over his body.

Theme: Cause of Neurological Symptoms

Options

A. Subarachnoid haemorrhage

B. Subdural haemorrhage

C. Extra dural haemorrhage

D. Intra cerebral haemorrhage

E. Multiple sclerosis

F. Intra cerebral abscess

G. Syphilis

H. Tuberculoma

I. Acute glaucoma

J. Stroke

Instructions

For each numbered item below, select the most appropriate answer from the options listed above. Each option may be selected once, more than once or not at all.

1135. A 72-year-old alcoholic with history of repeated falls presents with ataxia and headache.

1136. A rugby player was knocked down by bat and become unconscious but regained his consciousness quickly. But on the way to the hospital, he developed headache and comatose in the ambulance van.

1137. A 56-year-old woke up with hemiparesis of his right upper limb and dysphagia. After 4 hours, the symptoms subcided.

1138. A 45-year-old man develops sudden severe headache in the occiput.

1139. A 65-year-old male with history of hypertension, who didn't take any medication for the past 10 years presents with severe headache and right hemiplegia.

1140. A 56-year-old man presents with headache and while walking he is leaning towards left with instability.

ANSWERS

1	G	45	E	89	G	133	C
2	G	46	F	90	M	134	A
3	J	47	D	91	E	135	J
4	C	48	A	92	K	136	I
5	C	49	E	93	I	137	E
6	C	50	G	94	N	138	C
7	G	51	A	95	D	139	K
8	M	52	A	96	G	140	B
9	N	53	A	97	A	141	A
10	G	54	I	98	I	142	D
11	D	55	F	99	M	143	I
12	A	56	C	100	B	144	F
13	B	57	A	101	M	145	E
14	A	58	E	102	E	146	F
15	L	59	I	103	F	147	H
16	C	60	A	104	G	148	F
17	J	61	G	105	H	149	K
18	H	62	H	106	K	150	B
19	M	63	I	107	C	151	C
20	D	64	D	108	D	152	H
21	I	65	E	109	L	153	H
22	H	66	A	110	G	154	F
23	C	67	A	111	E	155	C
24	C	68	C	112	D	156	K
25	E	69	A	113	E	157	A
26	B	70	D	114	E	158	B
27	B	71	B	115	C	159	C
28	D	72	H	116	B	160	C
29	D	73	A	117	A	161	C
30	D	74	G	118	I	162	G
31	G	75	E	119	F	163	A
32	A	76	E	120	D	164	E
33	I	77	E	121	I	165	K
34	M	78	F	122	K	166	I
35	D	79	A	123	B	167	E
36	H	80	G	124	A	168	H
37	F	81	E	125	H	169	I
38	C	82	J	126	D	170	I
39	A	83	E	127	G	171	C
40	G	84	A	128	F	172	A
41	G	85	I	129	J	173	B
42	D	86	A	130	H	174	A
43	J	87	B	131	G	175	D
44	C	88	E	132	B	176	M

177 A	224 D	271 F	318 B
178 E	225 B	272 A	319 K
179 F	226 I	273 E	320 I
180 I	227 A	274 F	321 J
181 E	228 C	275 E	322 H
182 D	229 G	276 D	323 E
183 B	230 D	277 E	324 D
184 A	231 F	278 D	325 G
185 F	232 D	279 B	326 H
186 K	233 A	280 E	327 I
187 G	234 F	281 A	328 F
188 K	235 N	282 H	329 E
189 H	236 G	283 I	330 K
190 K	237 D	284 B	331 F
191 J	238 J	285 L	332 C
192 B	239 G	286 A	333 G
193 C	240 J	287 A	334 F
194 E	241 D	288 I	335 D
195 F	242 B	289 C	336 D
196 H	243 D	290 H	337 E
197 J	244 I	291 H	338 F
198 G	245 H	292 E	339 B
199 I	246 C	293 G	340 B
200 B	247 C	294 F	341 H
201 D	248 G	295 K	342 J
202 E	249 A	296 B	343 D
203 E	250 B	297 J	344 H
204 H	251 C	298 L	345 H
205 A	252 D	299 D	346 A
206 F	253 F	300 E	347 I
207 B	254 B	301 F	348 K
208 H	255 J	302 M	349 C
209 F	256 C	303 J	350 N
210 F	257 C	304 I	351 G
211 C	258 D	305 A	352 L
212 F	259 A	306 E	353 K
213 H	260 A	307 G	354 A
214 G	261 G	308 K	355 L
215 E	262 I	309 I	356 D
216 D	263 G	310 C	357 A
217 C	264 C	311 H	358 F
218 J	265 E	312 G	359 H
219 H	266 F	313 F	360 B
220 E	267 D	314 M	361 C
221 B	268 H	315 G	362 A
222 C	269 L	316 H	363 L
223 L	270 J	317 D	364 M

365 B	412 B	459 E	506 M
366 J	413 C	460 K	507 D
367 P	414 E	461 H	508 M
368 Q	415 G	462 E	509 G
369 G	416 D	463 A	510 G
370 K	417 J	464 D	511 B
371 G	418 J	465 F	512 A
372 J	419 E	466 D	513 E
373 A	420 D	467 C	514 F
374 F	421 D	468 H	515 C
375 C	422 G	469 T	516 D
376 B	423 H	470 F	517 F
377 L	424 I	471 E	518 J
378 D	425 F	472 G	519 I
379 H	426 B	473 B	520 K
380 A	427 A	474 M	521 G
381 C	428 I	475 0	522 F
382 H	429 C	476 J	523 D
383 J	430 H	477 I	524 A
384 A	431 E	478 F	525 J
385 E	432 K	479 G	526 M
386 K	433 E	480 E	527 F
387 K	434 D	481 H	528 J
388 J	435 J	482 L	529 I
389 0	436 F	483 M	530 K
390 J	437 A	484 E	531 J
391 D	438 E	485 M	532 M
392 G	439 J	486 A	533 H
393 A	440 H	487 C	534 E
394 C	441 F	488 B	535 M
395 C	442 C	489 B	536 A
396 F	443 K	490 F	537 A
397 D	444 J	491 I	538 G
398 M	445 B	492 L	539 D
399 D	446 F	493 D	540 C
400 I	447 E	494 C	541 F
401 A	448 I	495 G	542 C
402 H	449 K	496 E	543 B
403 A	450 I	497 B	544 M
404 G	451 F	498 A	545 E
405 J	452 B	499 P	546 F
406 H	453 D	500 F	547 G
407 K	454 C	501 I	548 F
408 A	455 A	502 B	549 K
409 D	456 F	503 L	550 C
410 B	457 D	504 G	551 A
411 C	458 B	505 A	552 I

553 C	600 G	647 C	694 B
554 I	601 B	648 F	695 A
555 N	602 G	649 X	696 C
556 F	603 F	650 H	697 D
557 K	604 A	651 G	698 L
558 B	605 C	652 S	699 0
559 E	606 H	653 0	700 G
560 B	607 F	654 K	701 E
561 0	608 C	655 H	702 B
562 A	609 K	656 B	703 A
563 A	610 J	657 M	704 C
564 D	611 K	658 0	705 D
565 M	612 H	659 0	706 L
566 L	613 M	660 B	707 0
567 D	614 L	661 L	708 G
568 F	615 N	662 G	709 C
569 P	616 A	663 A	710 P
570 P	617 F	664 I	711 G
571 A	618 D	665 B	712 C
572 B	619 B	666 B	713 F
573 J	620 J	667 M	714 K
574 C	621 B	668 L	715 B
575 G	622 B	669 G	716 D
576 F	623 E	670 L	717 P
577 E	624 B	671 A	718 A
578 N	625 P	672 C	719 A
579 E	626 E	673 I	720 I
580 F	627 C	674 K	721 0
581 K	628 F	675 K	722 A
582 B	629 C	676 K	723 D
583 D	630 H	677 T	724 E
584 I	631 E	678 I	725 G
585 L	632 G	679 F	726 G
586 P	633 I	680 B	727 K
587 A	634 J	681 D	728 H
588 F	635 E	682 C	729 K
589 G	636 B	683 A	730 A
590 J	637 F	684 H	731 D
591 C	638 E	685 N	732 K
592 D	639 B	686 D	733 I
593 H	640 H	687 E	734 E
594 I	641 F	688 B	735 C
595 K	642 D	689 C	736 D
596 K	643 M	690 A	737 A
597 0	644 L	691 D	738 A
598 E	645 E	692 E	739 K
599 I	646 J	693 H	740 C

741	B	788	C	835	A	882	E
742	F	789	B	836	E	883	C
743	A	790	F	837	C	884	G
744	B	791	A	838	A	885	F
745	A	792	I	839	K	886	F
746	F	793	C	840	B	887	D
747	B	794	D	841	C	888	G
748	K	795	F	842	I	889	B
749	A	796	C	843	I	890	D
750	G	797	G	844	D	891	E
751	D	798	B	845	H	892	C
752	F	799	A	846	E	893	A
753	C	800	C	847	F	894	A
754	E	801	B	848	G	895	B
755	C	802	D	849	B	896	D
756	C	803	G	850	C	897	G
757	A	804	E	851	C	898	A
758	D	805	B	852	G	899	B
759	G	806	G	853	H	900	E
760	A	807	F	854	B	901	C
761	A	808	F	855	B	902	A
762	J	809	B	856	I	903	H
763	F	810	A	857	I	904	J
764	I	811	C	858	C	905	A
765	A	812	A	859	D	906	E
766	B	813	E	860	E	907	G
767	C	814	D	861	C	908	D
768	H	815	B	862	C	909	A
769	G	816	D	863	A	910	E
770	A	817	A	864	F	911	B
771	C	818	C	865	B	912	E
772	C	819	Anti-D	866	H	913	F
773	F	820	F	867	B	914	E
774	D	821	D	868	I	915	C
775	l	822	C	869	J	916	A
776	E	823	B	870	C	917	E
777	D	824	D	871	D	918	B
778	F	825	H	872	K	919	D
779	E	826	C	873	A	920	F
780	B	827	J	874	G	921	G
781	A	828	F	875	J	922	E
782	C	829	B	876	C	923	M
783	A	830	C	877	E	924	N
784	G	831	H	878	G	925	A
785	F	832	R	879	F	926	K
786	G	833	E	880	A	927	G
787	C	834	B	881	B	928	H

929 N	976 M	1023 N	1070 D
930 G	977 L	1024 G	1071 A
931 C	978 A	1025 J	1072 F
932 J	979 F	1026 I	1073 A
933 H	980 E	1027 N	1074 D
934 F	981 I	1028 F	1075 A
935 L	982 A	1029 B	1076 E
936 N	983 E	1030 I	1077 E
937 K	984 F	1031 N	1078 D
938 F	985 J	1032 C	1079 C
939 J	986 L	1033 L	1080 A
940 B	987 C	1034 B	1081 L
941 A	988 B	1035 K	1082 A
942 E	989 M	1036 G	1083 C
943 F	990 K	1037 F	1084 F
944 K	991 M	1038 K	1085 G
945 L	992 G	1039 C	1086 E
946 M	993 L	1040 M	1087 A
947 I	994 D	1041 I	1088 B
948 D	995 A	1042 L	1089 G
949 G	996 H	1043 H	1090 G
950 F	997 K	1044 J	1091 A
951 I	998 B	1045 K	1092 F
952 J	999 F	1046 D	1093 G
953 A	1000 E	1047 A	1094 E
954 B	1001 D	1048 A	1095 B
955 K	1002 I	1049 H	1096 G
956 B	1003 A	1050 J	1097 C
957 H	1004 J	1051 F	1098 C
958 J	1005 B	1052 K	1099 A
959 C	1006 A	1053 A	1100 D
960 ?	1007 B	1054 F	1101 A
961 A	1008 C	1055 C	1102 H
962 N	1009 E	1056 C	1103 F
963 E	1010 N	1057 C	1104 I
964 B	1011 L	1058 A	1105 H
965 C	1012 C	1059 C	1106 D
966 H	1013 E	1060 F	1107 F
967 A	1014 I	1061 G	1108 F
968 D	1015 F	1062 I	1109 B
969 I	1016 E	1063 F	1110 B
970 K	1017 F	1064 A	1111 A
971 M	1018 K	1065 B	1112 H
972 L	1019 N	1066 C	1113 A
973 F	1020 M	1067 B	1114 H
974 E	1021 F	1068 G	1115 B
975 D	1022 H	1069 M	1116 F

1117 C	1123 E	1129 H	1135 B
1118 A	1124 I	1130 D	1136 C
1119 M	1125 B	1131 A	1137 E
1120 C	1126 D	1132 H	1138 A
1121 B	1127 C	1133 F	1139 J
1122 F	1128 A	1134 G	1140 G